DEADLY SPIN
A Kelly McKay Medical Thriller
Book 2 – Alaska

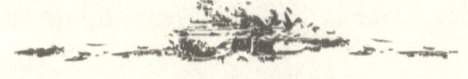

Betty Kuffel

DEADLY SPIN

Deadly Spin is a work of fiction. Events, setting, and characters are a work of imagination or are used fictitiously. You may recognize locations or characters similar to those in this novel, but they do not represent real places or people, nor do they suggest that the events described actually occurred.

OTHER TITLES BY AUTHOR

Deadly Pyre – A Kelly McKay Medical Thriller
Book 1 – Seattle

Coming Soon Kelly McKay Medical Thriller Series:

Deadly Crosswinds – Book 3 - Montana
Deadly Gold – Book 4 – Nevada

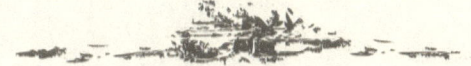

Alaska Flight – *A Romantic Medical Thriller*
Fatal Feast – *A Biological Thriller*

NONFICTION

Eyes of a Pedophile – *Detecting Child Predators*
True Crime
Your Heart – *Prevent & Reverse Heart Disease*
in Women, Men & Children
Modern Birth Control

Table of Contents

DEADLY SPIN

Chapter 1 Birdman

Crisscrossed restraints pinned a writhing young man face down on a stretcher. Medics and two police officers guided their patient toward waiting night staff in Anchorage Regional ER. A disheveled medic asked, "Where do you want him, Doc?"

"In lockdown." I pointed down a long hallway.

Vic's muscles strained his blue scrubs as the tall ex-military RN gripped the stretcher to help the medics roll it along. "I knew who it was when I heard your radio report. We haven't seen him for a while."

As ER doc for the night, I followed my next patient to a room where leather-cuffed straps dangled from a bed bolted to the floor. Grimy hands cuffed behind his back grabbed blindly at his captors. He spewed profanity and whipped his long hair from side to side as the entourage entered the room.

One of the police officers assisting the medics said, "This looks like a secure spot where he can't hurt anyone."

Vic eyed the unruly patient. "Yeah, except us."

I walked closer for a better look "I thought work in Alaska would be peaceful."

Vic told the group, "This is Dr. McKay's first week here on the job. She came from a trauma center in Seattle to relax."

"We wouldn't want you to get bored." An officer patted the patient's leg. "Tonight, this here nice man was making a disturbance at the Great Alaskan Bush Company, a topless joint downtown."

"The officers called us for backup." A medic at the patient's head spoke calmly. "You'll find a few bruises on Birdman. It took all of us to get him under control. He was screaming about the naked women shaking their boobies."

"I'll remove his cuffs when you're ready." An officer held up a key. "I've known him for years. He can be very nice, but this time he gets the wingnut of the week award."

Vic's six-three frame shielded me from the patient. "Let's calm him down before you get too close, Doc. Last time, he nearly broke a nurse's neck when he grabbed her hair." Vic directed the team, "We need to strip him and flip him onto the bed. We'll all be safer after he's locked in five-point leathers. I'm thinking we need two more guys to help us so nobody gets hurt."

The patient wailed. "Don't tie me down. Let me go and I'll get the hell out of here."

I said over the intercom, "We need two strong men to help us move a patient."

A voiced answered. "Security and Rob will be there in a minute."

Vic orchestrated the move. I'd helped manage violent patients many times during my training at Harbor Medical Center in Seattle, but I stood back and admired the former Marine in action. One look at Vic and most rowdy patients would do whatever he asked, but not this guy.

"Let's remove his jeans while he's still face down. Untie one leg at a time. Once he's undressed, wrap the leather cuffs around each ankle." Vic motioned to an officer. "I'll let you know when I'm ready to have you unlock his handcuffs. After that, you secure the waist belt, loop the cuffs, and attach each side to the bed frame.

While I waited out of reach, my anxiety rose just watching them.

"Dr. McKay, would you remove the spider straps when we have him under control?"

I nodded and moved closer.

Vic positioned himself at the patient's head. "I'll take the upper body. Rob, you take one arm, Security the other, a medic on each leg. On the count of three, we'll turn him over onto the bed and lock him to the frame."

Vic spoke in a calm voice. "John, you can make this easy on everyone, including yourself, by cooperating."

The patient screamed, "Go to hell!"

"If that's the way you feel, okay." Vic asked his cohorts, "Are you ready?"

In a valiant fight, John wrenched his torso free from Vic's grasp and kicked a medic. The patient's agitation and profanity spiked when his legs and body were fully restrained. Staff members vice-gripped his arms while Vic set about removing the man's turtleneck. He gave up when the patient clamped his chin down and then tried to bite him.

I hadn't expected such violence on my first night at work after moving to Alaska. I'd finished ER training three months earlier and recovered from near-fatal stab wounds. I say "recovered," but the sight of this violence clenched my gut and triggered anxiety I tried to suppress. Hiking and flying around the area had strengthened me and lowered my stress, but I wasn't quite ready for this.

Tonight, I had the urge to run.

Vic walked around to the patient's side and grabbed John's shirtfront. His muscles flexed beneath the blue scrubs as he twisted the fabric tight enough to stop the man's screams. Veins bulged on Vic's arms like the veins on the patient's purplish face and neck. "Hey, man, now that I've got your attention, listen to me." Vic said in a calm voice, "We're tryin' to help you. Now, cool it!" Vic shoved John into his pillow and let go of the shirt.

The patient's eyes flashed, and he spit.

Vic jumped back.

The cop ducked.

I wasn't fast enough. A big clot of sputum bypassed the men and stuck to my chest. I looked down at the slimy glob dangling off my left breast. My stomach convulsed.

I hate spit, but I had to laugh. Groans and snickers from the men joined me.

The patient's screams ceased. His eyes focused on my scrub top and then my face. "Why'd you get in the way, Dr. McKay? That was meant for the asshole muscleman."

How did this patient know me? He didn't look familiar.

Vic stood out of spitting range. "This is your doctor, John. Treat her with respect. No foul mouth. No more spitting."

The patient jerked at the restraints. "Please take these straps off, Dr. McKay. I'll leave peaceably."

"Sorry, I can't do that right now."

"Will you still take me flying, Doctor? Promise I'll behave."

Vic's eyes widened. "Do you know John?"

At first, I hadn't recognized him, but after his comment, panic surged again. "John Reilly, right?"

The patient nodded.

"We know each other from the Civil Air Patrol." I smiled at the disheveled man, hoping it would calm him if I spoke favorably. "We've searched for lost planes together. He volunteers at CAP like I do."

Vic looked incredulous. "You're shittin' me, Doc. We call him *Birdman* because of his incredible feather tattoos. I didn't know he was actually a flier."

With a smirk, a medic handed me some tissues. "Do you want me to help you, Doc?"

"Thanks for your thoughtfulness. I can tolerate blood, puke, and shit. Spit has made me throw up, but I think I can do this myself." I pulled off the projectile with a thick wad of tissue.

Vic explained. "Birdman is a paranoid schizophrenic. The voices screw with his thoughts when he doesn't take his meds." Experienced and blasé, Vic retrieved a syringe and small bottle from his scrub shirt pocket. He'd planned ahead after hearing the medic report. "Looks like a job for *vitamin H*. Birdman usually needs industrial doses. How much Haldol do you want?"

I said, "Start with five of Haldol, plus two of Ativan and fifty of Benadryl."

Vic smiled. "John usually needs more than a B-52, Doc. How about a C-5A?" He used the intercom. "I need two syringes of meds, stat. One with 2 milligrams of Ativan, the other with 50 milligrams of Benadryl." Vic pulled a dose of the antipsychotic drug Haldol into his syringe.

I spoke up. "Vic, I know those are types of military airplanes, but you got me when it comes to the drugs. I can see what I just ordered is a B-52, but what's a C-5A?"

"A helluva lot bigger airplane than a B-52. Carries more payload." He laughed at his own joke. "In addition to what you already ordered, I suggest we give five-milligram payloads of Haldol until he lands."

"New terminology, but the same drugs I like to use." Vic's size, confidence, and jokes eased my anxiety.

The two officers headed for the door. "We'd better get back on the street."

"Thanks, guys." I looked at the patient to see if he was listening. He was facing the opposite direction, so I wasn't sure. "I appreciate your background information on John."

"Yeah, thanks." Vic held up the syringe. "We could use your help holding him down for the injections before you leave."

John jerked at the restraints and yelled, "I hate those drugs! I want my lawyer. You can't tie me up. It's against the law. I'll sue you for assault."

A nurse arrived with the other drugs. Vic readied his tranquillizing darts. Flight nurse Rob, the policemen, a security guard, and two medics leaned across John. They held him while Vic took aim. Under the weight of the six men, John struggled and spit. Just before Vic stuck the patient's bare thigh with the needle, John wiggled a hand loose from a leather cuff and struck Rob, grabbing his flight suit shirt pocket.

The fabric ripped.

The team mashed down harder. Rob secured the restraint, and Vic jabbed his needle in to the hilt.

Rob examined the damaged pocket. "Damn. This is a new uniform."

I tried to place a mask over John's face to keep him from spitting at the crew members still holding him. He pulled away. "Hold still and stop spitting. Haldol will calm you down and stop the voices."

"The voices won't like it," John warned. "No drugs, Doc. Don't do it."

"You need medication to calm the voices. I don't want you to hurt anyone or yourself."

"That fucking stuff stops my brain."

Vic injected the next two meds into the man's thigh.

"You'll pay." John glared. "I'll remember what all of you have done to me."

Rob tightened the waist belt after checking the limb restraints to make sure they were tight enough but not inhibiting circulation. Five-point restraints—leathers around wrists, ankles, and waist—held John safely to the bed.

Vic pulled trauma shears from his pocket and chomped the dirty T-shirt up the front and along each sleeve. With it filleted open, we slid the clothing from beneath the man's back. Vic covered John with a warm blanket and suggested he rest.

I removed the mask and told John we'd be back after the sedatives took effect.

The door closed behind us and muffled John's cursing.

Down the hall, I sat at the nursing desk, periodically glancing at the silenced video screen as I read through John's thick medical record. Camera images showed his mouth moving, but the reduced audio volume blunted his tirade.

"Vic, you handled him well. This is not the same calm man who hung around the hangar washing airplanes and going on searches with me."

"I'm horrified you flew with him." Vic sat down beside me and touched my arm. "I've seen him stable on his meds but had no idea he was hanging around CAP. You are so lucky he didn't freak out on a flight."

"John gave me no reason to distrust him. Now, I feel like I'm invading his privacy by reading his life history."

"You'll have to get over that. You're his doctor and not his friend."

I wondered how I could have spent so many hours flying with John sitting in the right seat without picking up on his mental illness. "I enjoyed flying with him. A gentleman, good-looking, clean, nicely dressed. I wondered about the tattoos on his arms but never asked him."

"Wait till you see the ones on his back. He volunteers at the raptor center where they care for injured eagles and hawks." Vic explained, "He has a fixation on birds. On one of his many ER admissions, he said the voices in his head told him he could fly."

John Reilly's chart revealed numerous psychiatric hospitalizations for psychotic behavior. A year earlier, his discharge diagnosis read *paranoid schizophrenia with episodes of command hallucinations and delusions*. Reading on, I learned that his first psychotic break had occurred in college. He had earned his private pilot license and went to work for the Alaska Department of Fish and Game. After completing a biology degree with a 4.0 grade point average, he lost the pilot license due to a psychotic episode. Erratic behavior and failure to take his psychotropic medication resulted in him losing his job.

On his last admission, the note stated that John had sideswiped cars and rammed a building trying to evade unseen pursuers. They gave him 100 milligrams of injected Thorazine. The drug calmed his agitation but dropped his blood pressure so low he required fluid resuscitation.

I hoped he'd tolerate Haldol better than Thorazine.

Vic went in with me when I examined John twenty minutes later. His blood pressure remained normal, but he continued to slur threats and struggle against the restrains. "Since John's still fighting, let's give him five more of Haldol."

"I like the way you think, Doc. Soon, he'll rest like a baby." Vic pulled the vial from his shirt pocket and withdrew more liquid into a syringe.

"You might need some help."

"I think I can do it myself, but since you're willing, how about I hold him and you inject?" He handed me the syringe.

Vic placed one hand on John's knee and leaned forward to lock the leg I'd use for the injection against the bed.

I peered around Vic's muscles to look at the patient. "John, this is more medicine to keep you calm."

"Don't do it. I hate it. Please set me free." John didn't fight this time.

I jabbed the needle deep into a thigh muscle that tensed and then abruptly relaxed.

John appeared sad and resigned to the treatment. His voice was soft. "If my dad wasn't dead, he'd save me from you. He understood."

Stacked doses of antipsychotic and sedating drugs finally stopped his fighting. John's darting eyes slowed but still followed our movements. "John, are you calm enough now to cooperate? I'd like to help you."

"I don't need help, Doc—you do." He turned his face to the wall.

Intricate tattoos extended from his back, with furled finger-like feathers embracing his upper arms. Matted black curly hair obscured some of the green and black feathers. With drugs and restraints controlling him, John's bare chest rose and fell in slow breaths.

When I listened to his lungs and heart, John's eyes opened, glazed and partially hidden by long lashes. Black stubble darkened his attractive face. His heart rate quickened, then slowed. I pressed down on his belly to examine for abnormalities. His abdominal muscles twitched when my hand touched his sweaty skin. John moved toward me. His penis bulged beneath his shorts. Handcuff bruises encircled his wrists, now in leathers, holding his clenched fists secure. The young man's dirty body bore abrasions on the knees and elbows.

With John controlled by drugs, leather restraints, and Vic, I felt safe and was able to complete his exam. I talked to him in a calm voice. "I ordered a blood draw to check for some medical conditions. We also need a urine specimen for a drug screen. I want to see if there is any reason for your violent behavior, like PCP or methamphetamine. Do you use drugs?"

He didn't answer.

Vic rechecked John's blood pressure while I talked. "Is your violent behavior from drugs, or is your brain playing tricks on you again?"

"No drugs." He shook his head. "My brain shorts out sometimes, like my Mom's used to."

The meds softened John's threatening glares. "130 over 90. That's a good blood pressure, John. Probably better than mine right now."

Vic helped the lab tech. John didn't resist the tech's needle.

John's psychiatric evaluation correlated with his history of violent behavior related to disordered thoughts. I would never again be able to trust him enough to fly with me. What would I do if he went crazy and took the controls? "Would you call and see if they have a bed for him at API, Vic?"

Vic picked up the phone and made transfer arrangements to Alaska Psychiatric Institute.

"I hate that place, Doc. They lock me up with nut cases and expect me to get better. I'll be out in a couple days if I say the right things in group therapy and take their damn pills." John's words were slurred, but he was right.

I walked out of the room feeling his eyes on me.

Medications further dulled John's senses as we watched him on the video monitor and waited for his transfer. One of the nurses commented, "I like our new spy cameras. It's easier to keep a close eye on patients, but the cameras also provide better security at night."

Vic explained, "We got more assaults and drug problems when Anchorage grew rapidly during the pipeline boom. The ER got downright ugly." Vic pointed to Room 1. "We had a bar fight continue in there. A gun-toter fired off a round." His words sent a flash of adrenaline to my brain.

"We had a knife fight in Harbor ER but never had shots fired."

"That shot shattered the ambulance door and triggered a meeting between police and hospital administration."

Flight nurse Rob, who'd been listening to our conversation, broke out laughing. "Right after that, administration hired more guards and installed surveillance cameras everywhere. Should I tell Kelly about Big Brother watching us?"

Vic smiled. "Go ahead."

"Now they video everything. Nose picking. Scratching unmentionable places, and trysts in the parking garage. We've all been more careful since they caught Dr. Wells and a nurse doin' the wild thing on video."

A female RN said, "Served him right. His wife used the video against him in the divorce."

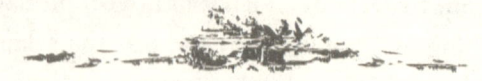

A couple hours after John Reilly's arrival, the same medics who had wheeled him in wheeled him out. They drove the somnolent Birdman to the confines of Alaska Psychiatric Institute, where a tall concertina wire-topped fence surrounded the austere brick structure housing the depressed, psychotic, and legally insane of Alaska.

Chapter 2 An Alaska Friend

At 11:30 p.m., the phone line for medical helicopter transport rang. Flight nurse Rob Lewis answered on the first ring and listened for a moment and then handed me the phone. "Dr. McKay, Palmer Hospital ER needs us to transport a cardiac. Dr. Gordon is on the line. I'll call our pilot to check weather and see if it's a go."

I spoke into the receiver. "Kelly McKay, here. I'm ER doc tonight. What's going on?"

"Oh, Kelly, hello. I have a challenge for you."

"I hear you always do." I smiled, recalling some of the train-wreck stories my cohort Lynn, another ER doctor from Seattle and the one who had lured me to Anchorage, had told me. The skilled old physician worked in a rural area on the edge of disaster. The small hospital, located an hour's drive or a twenty-minute flight from Anchorage, transferred many patients to Regional ER.

"This one's an unstable cardiac. A wonderful old dog musher I've known for years. Despite his crushing chest pain, Ed drove himself here to Palmer from his home in Wasilla. We dragged him out of his truck onto a stretcher and into ER, sweaty and weak."

The doctor drawled on in a Texas accent. "Ed's EKG showed *tombstone* ST elevations, probably occluding his LAD. I cooled him off with oxygen, nitroglycerine, and morphine. His pain's gone." He paused for a few seconds. I heard muffled words in the background before he returned. "Be damned if the EKG didn't just normalize. I called a few minutes ago and consulted Smoky Severson, your cardiologist on call tonight. He accepted Ed in transfer. Is the helicopter available?"

"Rob is checking with the pilot. Great work on Ed. You saved another one."

"Mostly luck. I've got blood thinners going."

"Good. Your patient needs a quick trip to the cath lab."

"Sure does. Smoky will fix him up."

I watched Rob talking on the phone to our pilot. He nodded to me and circled his finger overhead imitating a helicopter rotor.

To Dr. Gordon, I said, "They'll be taking off in a few minutes. Call me if anything changes."

"Thanks, Kelly." The GP sounded relieved. "We'll be listening for the ship." He sucked in a noisy breath. "His wife, Lucille, and a couple dogs came along for the ride. She called a friend to drive her to Anchorage. I sure hope Ed makes it."

Rob and a flight EMT rushed out to the helicopter. Soon, thudding blades shook windows as it lifted off and disappeared into the night.

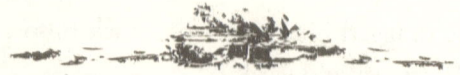

We had nearly cleared the ER of patients by the time the radio crackled to life with a report from the inbound med flight. "Regional ER, this is Lifeguard."

I answered. "Regional ER, go ahead."

"We have a 70-year-old male on board with an acute MI. His pain recurred en route." Radio silence for a moment. "He's on a heparin drip and just started throwing PVCs. Is the cath lab ready?"

"They're here and waiting. Give him some morphine. We'll be on the pad to give you a hand. What's your ETA?"

"Less than ten minutes."

I went outside with an RN and Dr. Severson. We waited near the landing pad, scanning the clear Alaskan night sky. The chain-smoking cardiologist stepped away from us and lit up in air so still the smoke clung like fog around him, providing both first- and secondhand smoke. Smoky was a skilled cardiologist with a bad habit. Vic told me Smoky could talk someone into quitting smoking with a cigarette in each hand but couldn't quit himself.

The sound of helicopter blades grew louder. Red/green position lights bore down on us from the northeast like a spaceship.

Smoky cleared his throat and moved closer. "It was supposed to be twenty degrees tonight. I think it's colder."

"It's too cold to stay out here without a coat." I went back inside to escape the cold and the trailing smoke. Rob's voice from the helicopter came in over the base station radio at the desk. "His pain is back. Blood pressure is 80. I'm bolusing him with saline. Break." Radio silence. "He just went into third-degree block with wide complexes, rate 30 for a few beats. Now it's back at a rate of 90. I have pacer patches on him."

The helicopter touched down, and the crew whisked the patient inside. They moved down the hall toward the cath lab ahead of the patient's wheezing doctor, who struggled to keep up while getting a medical history from the patient. I hurried with them, watching the portable heart monitor and the old man's ashen face. Crow's-feet at the edges of his milky blue eyes deepened. A little smile appeared on his pale lips.

I smiled back. "How's the pain, Ed?"

"It's getting better again, honey. The doc in Palmer said a beautiful lady doctor with curly red hair would meet me. It has to be you."

"It is. I'm Kelly McKay."

"Dr. Kelly, I have a lot of mushing to do. Get me through this and I'll teach you to race sled dogs. Come out to visit when I'm feeling better." Gnarled fingers clutched his chest. "My wife Lucille makes the best bread on earth. A friend's drivin' her here. Would you tell her I'm gonna be okay?"

"I'll watch for them and keep her informed."

His smile changed to a grimace, and the stretcher disappeared into the lab.

I walked slowly back to ER. How could someone make me care so much after knowing him for about one minute? An LAD occlusion could take out half the heart. I hoped he'd survive.

Because Lucille hadn't arrived by the time my shift ended, I called the Palmer hospital to see if she had left yet and to give the doc out there a patient report.

His voice answered after four rings.

"Hi, it's Kelly. What are you doing answering the phone?"

"We're a little staffed. The nurse just ran to OB to help my partner with a delivery. I'm manning the phones and the ER while she's gone."

"I hope you get to go home and sleep soon."

He laughed. "I slept a couple hours on the job before Ed got here, so I'm okay for a while."

"That's good. Ed made it to the cath lab. En route here, his pain returned, and he had an episode of heart block. Has Lucille left yet?"

"They should be there in half an hour. Don't know how she'd make it without him. Lucille runs the house and Ed does everything else."

"I already like him. I'm off duty, but I'll wait for Lucille. Dr. Severson may be done with his stent by the time she gets here."

"That's nice of you to stay. They are great people."

"In the middle of a heart attack, he invited me to go mushing."

"I'm not surprised. He devotes his energy to raising and training sled dogs while she does the cooking and keeps him in line."

"They sound like hardy Alaskan types."

"Lucille looks frail, but she's tough as nails. Used to be a card dealer in Reno."

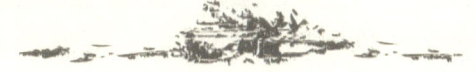

I walked to the cath lab monitor suite, where I sat in the semidarkness and watched a small tube snake inside Ed's coronary artery and spurt radiopaque dye. The video image showed a high-grade obstruction of the large coronary artery on the front of the heart. A balloon near the tip of the catheter inflated. The blocked area expanded. On another monitor screen, the electrocardiogram rhythm abruptly changed from the squiggle indicating heart injury to a burst of rapid, wide electrical complexes. A cath tech noted the sudden change. "V-tach! We've got V-tach!"

"Shock him!" Smoky ordered. "Cough, Ed, cough."

Sometimes a sharp cough converts the abnormal rhythm. Techs pressed the charge button and waited.

Groggy from the meds they'd given him, Ed came out of his fog and coughed. It didn't work. The wide lethal rhythm persisted, and he lost consciousness.

The cath team stepped away from the table, gloved hands held away from their bodies. A nurse applied defibrillator paddles to Ed's chest and pressed the button.

Ed's body convulsed.

The monitor image went flatline.

I held my breath.

A normal rhythm emerged and marched across the screen.

Smoky squirted more dye. He turned to see me observing the show and gave a thumb up. Through his mask he called, "Kelly, we've got good flow now. Other than a little V-tach arrest, he's doing great. Next, I've got to get the stent in."

I went to the waiting room and found a miniature woman with deep wrinkles. Strands of poufy gray hair escaped from pink plastic combs that matched her wool cardigan. Dressed in black polyester pants and a purple turtleneck shirt, her arthritic hands clung to the bottom of her sweater as she paced in the small room.

A tense man in his twenties wearing tattered Carhartt overalls and a black and red wool shirt with elbow patches sat on the edge of a chair. He stood when I entered and placed his arm around Ed's wife, braced for the worst.

"Hello. I'm Dr. McKay. Are you Lucille?"

She nodded. In a gravelly voice, she asked, "How's the old man doin'?"

"He's doing great. Dr. Severson is still working on him. He opened the blocked heart artery and is putting in a stent to keep it open. The doctor in Palmer did a good job getting him here so fast."

Lucille smiled. "Dr. Gordon is old as the hills, just like us. We love him. Thanks, Doctor." Lucille turned to the young man. "This is our good friend, Al Powers." She looked up at the tall man. "He's been helping Ed take care of the dogs." She smiled lovingly. "He's like the son we never had."

I shook her hand and then his. "Good to meet both of you. Could I get some coffee while you wait?"

"Black for both of us," Al responded. "Too bad we don't have one of those sticky buns you made yesterday, Lucille. Man, those were tasty."

I laughed. "As sick as Ed was when he was wheeled in here, he told me you make great bread."

Tears spilled from her worried eyes and tracked down the deep grooves in her cheeks. "Please come out and have some when Ed gets home. You can meet the dogs, too. We have seventy of them and some new puppies."

I worried Ed might not make it home.

Chapter 3 Life in Alaska

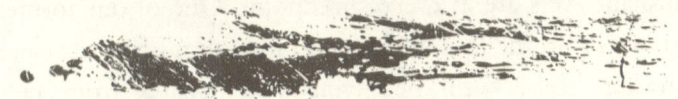

I walked the few blocks home to an apartment I shared with my good friend Lynn Cabot, the other ER doctor from Seattle. A brilliant sun sparkled on the hoarfrost coating tree branches against a cloudless sky. Snow crunched with each footstep. The Chugach Mountain Range facing Anchorage in the east stood in stark contrast against the blue backdrop. Jagged white summits commanded the skyline.

Neither Lynn nor I were great housekeepers, but she was worse. I entered the apartment and surveyed the mess of dirty dishes and strewn clothing. She was due back from a three-day snowmobile outing with Dale Ayers, chief pilot of our medical flight program. I should have cleaned the place but decided to get some sleep instead.

With bedroom windows covered by aluminum foil taped tight to keep out all light, I snuggled beneath my down comforter in the blackness and listened to radio news about the Iditarod racers. Even though this was my first winter in Alaska, dog racing had piqued my interest. But meeting Ed made me wonder how anyone could love dogs so much they'd own seventy of them.

The announcer reported: "The mushers left Anchorage five days ago. They travel by the light of headlamps and the moon. Right now, along the trail to Nome, it's snowing and drifting the trail shut. Visibility is bad. A few mushers have dropped out. Others are holed up waiting for conditions to improve. On the lighter side, there are no reported dog mishaps. Vets are at every checkpoint. One of our former winners is in the lead, with three of last year's finalists close on her heels. We'll be giving you updates from race headquarters as we receive them."

I pinched yellow foam plugs and stuffed them in my ears before turning off the radio. White noise from a fan blunted the daytime sounds as I fell asleep.

In late afternoon, I awakened to the smell of bacon and Dale's obnoxious laugh. I cracked open my bedroom door. Lynn stood in the kitchen frying eggs. Her snowsuit, boots, helmet, and mitts lay in a heap near the door. Dale sat on the couch with stockinged feet on the coffee table. He was slamming down a beer. An empty can lay on its side near his feet.

I wondered how long they'd been home. Wearing a bulky robe, I plopped down beside Dale and immediately knew I'd chosen a bad spot to sit. His rank body odor after three days without a shower clouded the air. "Hi, you two, I heard Dale's laugh and smelled the bacon."

Lynn turned away from the stove. "Hi, Kelly. Sorry if we woke you."

My eyes widened. "Lynn, what happened to your face?"

"I fell off the snow machine on a steep grade and did a face plant. I rolled about twenty feet down the hill, the machine ahead of me. That's what Dale was laughing about."

"That doesn't sound very funny. You could have been killed."

"I'm okay. I'd removed the face mask from my helmet because it was too warm. The hard snow scratched my face and packed around my neck. I didn't get hurt much, but I look like Dale beat me up, don't I?"

"You're right." I walked to the kitchen. "What are you fixing? I'm starved."

"Just bacon and a fried egg sandwich for each of us. Do you want one?"

"Yes. Do I have time to shower and dress?"

"If you hurry. I'll fix your egg last."

I returned with wet hair, nearly ready to leave for work.

Dale sat at the table with a third beer in hand. "Has my crew been flying?"

"Last night we had a flight to Palmer for a cardiac, but it's been quieter than usual."

Lynn served the food and coffee. "On our trip, Dale told me tales of his work as a helicopter logger in southeast Alaska and in the military." She leaned over and kissed his gray beard. "Flying for us in the wilds of Alaska is easy compared to what he's been through."

"I'm glad you've had so much experience. A medical program like this carries a lot of responsibility." I watched Dale guzzle. How Lynn could actually like him was beyond comprehension.

Lynn, a rich Bostonian, seemed out of place in Alaska, but why was she with this old redneck Alabaman? She had left neurosurgeon Neville Carrington behind in Seattle. He was needy but a gentleman. She wanted to escape from her roots and her society parents. Mission accomplished.

Lynn served us the food and coffee. Dale's self-satisfied smile changed to a beer-fumed belch.

Lynn laughed. "Didn't your mother teach you any manners, Dale?"

"Nope. She ran off when I was in diapers. My pappy raised me. Learned my manners from him."

I was happy to leave Dale behind when I set out in winter darkness for the hospital a few blocks away. At work, I took care of a couple of patients with minor problems and sneaked away to visit Ed. He waved and strolled down the hall toward me with a monitor battery-box weighing down the pocket of his long robe. "Dr. Kelly, I go home tomorrow. No heart damage. I'm a walking advertisement for the latest plumbing techniques."

"Great news. You're looking good."

"I feel better than I have in weeks. This must have been coming on and I didn't realize it. I felt real short of breath out in the cold but just thought I was getting old." We sat on a couch in an alcove. "I want you to meet the dogs. Can you come out on your next day off? If you call ahead, Lucille will have a meal ready."

"I'll come out soon. Is it easy to find your place?"

"Just watch the mile markers on the Parks Highway past Wasilla. We live near Nancy Lake. You can't miss it."

"I have to get back to ER now. I'll call soon. Take care. Hug the dogs for me."

His blue eyes twinkled. "Okay, honey. Thanks for everything."

Back in ER, Rob Lewis asked, "So, how's the old musher?"

"Up walking and pain-free. Severson told him he had no heart damage. He sounded sincere about me coming out to visit."

"Take him up on it. Visiting a dog farm is part of the Alaskan experience. He must have liked you on sight. Here he was having the big one, and he hustled you on his way into the cath lab."

"He's a nice old guy. I usually hate it when people call me *honey*, but, coming from Ed, I actually liked it. He's like a grandfather."

"Ed's famous for raising the smartest, sweetest, best-trained dogs around. Many have run the Iditarod. He used to win sprint races in his younger days."

"He said he'd teach me to run dogs."

"Watch out or you'll have a team of your own. He'll be giving you puppies you can't resist." Rob turned up the radio. "Your temporary assignment will become permanent, and you'll be running the big race."

"Not a chance. I really like being warm when I sleep."

Rob laughed. "Mark my words."

The small radio gave us a commentary on the race's progress while I sat in the nursing station writing admission orders on a man with pneumonia, a three-pack-a-day smoker.

About 3 a.m., the police scanner alerted us to a domestic with shots fired. The call came from Spenard, a poor area near the international airport. Being isolated and living in poverty during the long winter darkness brought out the worst in people. An ambulance stood by, waiting to be cleared to enter the trailer house. The ER staff listened to the radio wondering if we'd be getting a patient.

Within a few minutes, an excited medic reported, "En route code 3, with one. Thirty-year-old female, agonal. Gunshot wound to the left chest. Tubed and getting a line in. CPR in progress. ETA six minutes."

Rob said, "That's the third Spenard divorce this winter."

"What do you mean?" The nurses liked to tease me with local jargon.

"We get a lot of people with cabin fever in the wintertime. Lack of daylight takes its toll. Tempers flare, and too much alcohol adds to the problem. Everyone carries a gun, and somebody gets shot."

Another nurse added, "It happens all the time. Even judges get complacent. Watch the newspaper. Last year, one guy who shot his wife was out on bail, while another guy who killed a moose out of season went to jail."

We met the ambulance at the door and rushed the injured woman into a large trauma room equipped like an operating room. Bright lights, X-ray, monitors, suction, and oxygen stood ready.

One glance told me she was dead. Her skin was a transparent white due to blood loss.

Rob, a flight nurse, and Vic, the former Marine, had O negative blood ready to give her. I shook my head.

The medic continued pumping on her chest. "Dr. McKay, there was a lot of blood at the scene. No cardiac activity."

"What caliber gun?"

The medic lifted his hand for me to see her chest. ".357, left chest, below the nipple."

A dark hole with purple edges. I checked her eyes, listened to her lungs as the medic squeezed the oxygen bag, and felt for a pulse with the compressions. "Did you look at her exit wound?"

He nodded. "It's big and left a pool of blood on the floor. I slapped on a pad to seal the bleeding site. We tubed her, loaded, and ran."

"Hold CPR. Turn her quickly for me to look at the exit site." I helped turn her body.

The second medic said, "Don't know how long it was between the time she was shot and when the police were able to get us in there. At least ten minutes with no respiratory effort and no pulse. Her pupils were fixed and dilated."

Her back told us why. She had a gaping three-inch-diameter hole exposing lung tissue and bone fragments near her spine.

"Stop resuscitation." I looked at the wall clock. "We'll call it at zero-three-twenty."

A pale, sweaty medic said, "We should have left her at the scene. It looked futile from the start, but there were three crying kids. It was just awful."

"You did the right thing to transport her under those circumstances."

"The police will be here, but they were trying to deal with the husband. He kept claiming she shot herself. A little girl about seven screamed, 'Daddy shot Mommy, Daddy shot Mommy!' She hugged her little brother and sister, two of the cutest little buggers you'd ever see. Her little arms were so skinny." His voice trembled. "I have kids about the same age."

After looking closer at the entrance wound, I left the room. The bullet had tracked through the chest front to back, through both lungs at an angle. Based on the trajectory, the position of the exit wound made it unlikely she had shot herself, whether she was right- or left-handed.

Vic called the coroner.

My next patient had a toothache. He fished for narcotics and information. "I've been listening to your scanner. You got some real excitement around here tonight, just like on TV. I got friends in Spenard. What's her name? Maybe I know her."

"Sorry, I can't tell you. You'll have to read about it in the newspaper. Tell me about your dental problem."

"I got bad teeth. Rotted off to the roots. Usually, they don't hurt, but tonight my jaw swelled up and the pain is bad."

I examined his mouth and found a recurring medical and social problem I'd seen a lot of in Seattle. A few snags remained. Tonight's trouble stemmed from a brownish lump bathed in pus surrounded by swollen tissue.

"I think you need a dentist to pull the rest of your teeth. They're in bad shape."

"Can't afford it. They want money in advance."

Same old story. An ER had to treat anyone who showed up. Dentists didn't. I wished more dentists would provide gratis care. "Well, tonight I'll give you antibiotics and pain medicine. It will get you through the problem temporarily, but you have to see a dentist. If you get worse, come back to the ER."

"I will, Doc. Give me something strong. Had bleedin' ulcers so can't take them Motrins. I took two of my friend's Percocets to make it here. I'm feeling a little better. Thanks for helpin' me."

Rob returned with a starter pack of meds and discharged the man. He followed me back to the desk where Vic sat talking to the coroner. "Kelly, you should learn to pull teeth. You'd be a busy lady. These night prowlers with dental problems would refer all their friends to you. Was it like that in Seattle, too?"

"The same, but a minor problem compared to the volume of trauma. I don't miss Seattle at all. The gunshot wound tonight reminded me how good we have it. You don't have many really bad things come through here, do you?"

Vic answered. "True but seeing that poor woman dead and leaving behind three little kids is hard to take. ER and the military can ruin you, if you let it. We all have to take the time to live." His penetrating blue eyes searched my face. "Have you been playing since you arrived in Anchorage?"

"Not much. I've been studying for the Boards. The test is next month. During the fall, I hiked, and I flew with the Civil Air Patrol."

Vic leaned close enough that I could feel his warmth, emotionally and physically. He was likeable and sexy, but after my bad choice of men in the past, I was afraid to let him penetrate my barrier. "You looked a little spooked by that psychotic guy we had a few nights ago."

"I thought I'd recovered from the knife attack, but some things trigger my anxiety when I least expect it."

"I recognized your reaction. I'm strong as an ox, but a few things happened in the Marines that stayed with me. One day a buddy sneaked up behind me. I knocked him flat. It just came out of nowhere. Shocked me more than him." Vic smiled gently. "We'll take care of you, Doc. Don't worry."

I'd only been around for a few months, but I felt like I had better friends here than I'd ever had in my life. "Thanks, Vic. I hate feeling like a wimp."

Maybe I'd change my mind about men, at least about Vic. I might like having him take care of me.

Chapter 4 A Lost Musher

Lynn dragged herself into ER, late for the 7 a.m. shift, and collapsed into a chair near the desk. If I hadn't known better, I would have thought she was a victim of domestic abuse. Her wavy blond hair framed facial bruises partially hidden beneath makeup. She brightened after drinking the cup of coffee I handed to her before I started my report and handoff of patients.

"Thanks for the coffee. I'm more awake, but I'd like to go back to bed and sleep till noon."

I finished the report on two remaining patients and then slipped on my down jacket. "Sunrise is my favorite time of day. I like getting up early or walking home after a night shift."

"Kelly, you're sick. We're exact opposites. I hate it when you're filled with energy and cheerful in the morning. I don't see how anyone can be like that."

"You're just tired after the trip."

"I'm tired, but more upset than anything. Dale and I had some nasty arguments." Her hand shook as she brought the cup to her mouth. "He drank too much and took routes the other two couples thought were avalanche risks. Still, I had a wonderful time."

"I was surprised he drank four beers before I left for work last night. I don't think I've ever been with you two when he wasn't drinking."

"He is a real man, not like those prissy Easterners I used to date. I grant you, he's a little rough on the edges. I'm working on that, but he was upset over the fight with his friends and me." Lynn stiffened. "And don't start harping on his drinking. He drank nothing after you left. Be quiet when you go in. He's asleep on the couch."

"Code blue, cardiac arrest in ICU" repeated overhead. Lynn ran to the code.

I trudged the icy sidewalk along the five-block route to our apartment.

A dusting of snow covered the ice and made walking treacherous. I grabbed a bush to right myself after a near fall. I looked up to see two moose rounding a corner and tromping down the sidewalk a few feet from me. They were bigger than horses and made no move to change course. I scrambled over a snowbank and stood between two parked cars to let them pass.

The moose stopped and examined me with large brown eyes so close I saw their pupils constrict in the bright sun. Their exhalations puffed fog into icy air and turned to frost on their funny faces. Glistening crystals clung to their lashes. The animals looked like goofy cartoon characters, but I'd read about unsuspecting humans and dogs who were trampled to death by these unique creatures clinging to a wild existence in an urban world.

Orange Fish and Game radio collars monitored their travels. They ambled toward the hospital, stopping to nibble on shrubs. Once they passed me, I tracked in the opposite direction.

Dale was gone from the apartment, and I felt relieved. I cleaned up dishes, threw a load of clothes in the washer, and set the alarm for noon so I wouldn't waste my three days off. I planned to call Ed and make sure he was home and doing well.

At 11 a.m., the phone rang. I recognized Dale's voice. "Sorry to wake you, but Lynn told me you're off work for the next couple days. I need an observer to go on a long Civil Air Patrol search with me. There's a lost musher."

"I'll go if you'll be doing the flying. I've only had about three hours of sleep." Dale sounded alert. It had been more than twelve hours since his last drink, so he met the "8 hours from bottle to throttle" FAA safety regulation regarding alcohol consumption.

"Good, I'm glad you're willing to join me. The musher went through McGrath and made it past Cripple Creek. He didn't show up at Ruby. Visibility along the route is poor due to blowing snow. Weather is good enough for us to make it to the search base at McGrath. I'll pick you up in fifteen minutes."

"Are you bringing food?"

"I have dried food packs and snacks left over from the snow cat trip. Bring survival gear, sleeping bag. and an overnight kit. I don't know when we'll be back. Dress warm. I'll buy you lunch at Peggy's Cafe before we leave."

After a quick hot shower, I dressed in layers. Silk long underwear topped with wool long johns, polar fleece pants, and then wool pants. Two pairs of socks, a turtleneck, and a wool sweater. I brought a hooded down jacket, a sleeping bag, a lightweight foam pad, and a fanny pack with two energy bars, a water bottle, and a toothbrush.

I put my gear by the door. When he rang the doorbell, I opened it immediately.

Dale jumped back. "You startled me. Other than wet hair, Kelly, looks like you're ready." He laughed. "I'm impressed. I was gonna put a little pressure on you by arriving early. You and Lynn are cool women. None of that prissy stuff with hot rollers."

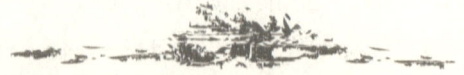

I strapped on my double-clip 9-millimeter Smith and Wesson and a Buck folding knife, both necessary survival gear in Alaska. I'd also taken to carrying an emergency Bic lighter even though I don't smoke. These were all items I carried in the plane when I flew.

We climbed into Dale's Ford Explorer, which looked more like a garbage truck than an SUV. The back seat was heaped with dirty clothes from an overturned basket, apparently en route to the laundromat. Wadded up fast-food wrappers strewed the floor. I placed my gear on top of his flat spare tire.

As I cinched my seat belt, Dale drove too fast over icy roads to Peggy's Cafe on the other side of town. The restaurant sat across the street from the east-west runway at Merrill Field, near the CAP hangar. The landmark place, painted lavender and ugly as hell on the exterior, was filled with jovial fliers and local color eating large greasy meals and great pie.

Dale and I sat down at the first available table, next to a table for six filled with men wearing press badges and down jackets so new I looked for tags. Dale pulled off his hat, exposing unruly gray stick-straight hair. He didn't even bother to finger-comb it.

A bearded man at the table wearing a wool plaid shirt nodded hello to Dale.

I whispered, "Who's that? He looks familiar."

"Our governor. I think he's on a publicity tour."

Dale and I stripped off our warm tops and hung them on the chair backs.

One of the pressmen watched me pulling my wool sweater off over my head. His eyes fixated on the handgun at my waist.

I smiled sweetly.

He said something to the governor.

The governor nodded our way. "I don't think you have to worry about her shooting you. I bet they are going on a search. Hey, Dale, where are you and the lady headed? My New York guests are a bit threatened by the hardware you're wearing."

"There's an overdue musher out past McGrath. We're joining the aerial search. Others are searching along the trail on snow machines."

"Hadn't heard. Hope he's okay."

"He'd been in the top ten, but after a storm blew in, he didn't show up at Ruby." Dale scanned the menu. "Once we get a load of cholesterol, we'll be heading out. The weather between here and there doesn't look too bad."

"Good luck. We're all going to Unalakleet and, in a couple days, on to Nome to watch the finish."

Dale turned back to me. "That's what I like about Alaska. You even get to know the governor on a first-name basis. He's a real Alaskan, not one of those politician types."

"I like Alaska, too. Big and desolate but flying makes it all come together. I want to buy a plane before summer, so I can get out to see more of the country."

Dale raised his eyebrows. "Do you have your taildragger endorsement?"

"No, but I plan to get it this spring when the weather warms up. It's too much of a hassle to dig a plane out of the snow to fly for a couple hours of training."

"The flight school will do it for you. I'd recommend you start now. You'll be confident by the time you're serious about putting your money down. Are you thinking of tricycle gear or taildragger?"

"I've been watching Trade-A-Plane and cruising the flight line at Merrill looking at For Sale signs." I'd looked at many planes, but none seemed perfect for me. "I think I want one that will get me way out, out to the small bush strips and maybe even sandbars. A real Alaskan airplane."

"The Maule is a strong, dependable taildragger. You could carry the kitchen sink in it, if that's one of your criteria."

"I flew a Maule with an instructor in Washington. But, I like Super Cubs for their versatility."

"It's like buying a truck. Get the right one for the job."

A couple of old duffers at another table cut in. "So, the little lady wants to buy a taildragger? That can be a lot of airplane to handle in a crosswind."

I smiled.

One old guy said, "Make sure you get a good one and fly only in fair weather. We lose a bunch of airplanes every year because those flatlanders from Outside come up here and don't realize Alaska's unforgiving."

Dale took a bite and spoke as he chewed. "I'll make sure she gets a good plane and the right training. She's got brains and won't push the weather."

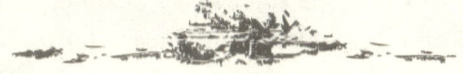

A squeaky metal door with a small security window provided entry to the Civil Air Patrol hangar. A ten-foot-long Formica table on metal legs sat on a cement floor covered with worn linoleum in the pilots' lounge. Rickety metal folding chairs surrounded it. A sign that said "No Smoking Allowed" hung on the wall over an overflowing garbage can reeking of cigarette ashes and oily pepperoni pizza boxes. The combined smells after my sausage and egg breakfast knotted my stomach and surged acid into my throat. I hoped we wouldn't run into turbulence on the flight.

We walked through the lounge into a large hangar housing many planes. The briefing window guarded a small room filled with radios, microphones, a tiny TV, and a large, older ex-military man with an outdated crewcut. Cecil sat with his back to the window, perspiring in his short-sleeved plaid shirt. Two fat rolls along the base of his skull resembled kielbasa. When the jolly hard-working volunteer heard us at the window, he spun around with a big smile on his face.

"Hi, Dale. Thought you'd be here soon. Good to see you, Dr. Kelly." Cecil got up and stood at the window. "I have the twin ready for you, the 310. The mechanic just finished its annual check, so it shouldn't give you any trouble." He handed Dale the key. "Wing covers are in the rear baggage compartment. Weather guessers are reporting a six-thousand-foot ceiling and light snow along your route."

"Thanks for getting everything ready for us. We'll do a quick walk-around, check the oil, and be airborne."

"You have full fuel. Give me position and weather reports when you can so I can keep our other pilots updated. Still no word on the musher. We have two other planes up there on the search, along with locals in ski-planes."

The radio crackled alive with communication between Merrill Tower and an inbound student pilot doing pattern work. After hearing Cecil's weather forecast, I'd have rather stayed in Anchorage than fly cross-country. Flying in Alaska carried risk, and weather worsens without warning.

Cecil was one of the first fliers I met when I moved to Anchorage. CAP allowed me to fly on searches without expense. I volunteered my time to help search for people and in the process gained experience. I hoped we wouldn't need his luck and waved back. I commented to Dale, "Cecil looks sick."

"I agree. I thought maybe you knew. He had a bad heart attack last year before you moved here and can't fly anymore. Flying was his life, so he's dealing with depression."

"All of his experience makes him a skilled coordinator. I flew on some searches during the summer with him in charge and liked his manner and organization."

"Cecil's a dedicated radioman. He understands what we're up against out there and, like us, takes his volunteer job seriously."

My confidence flying with Dale over isolated snow-covered land improved as I walked with him around the plane. He performed the preflight checklist on the large twin-engine plane with care. When he finished, I pushed a button to open the huge hangar door.

Dale moved the Cessna outside with a motorized tug. After he parked the tug back inside, I lowered the door and followed him to the plane. He strapped himself into the left-hand seat and adjusted his headset. For an adequate view forward and to reach the controls, I positioned two cushions on the copilot's seat. I'd flown with Dale on other searches and appreciated the instruction he provided, allowing me to take off and fly to gain more experience at the controls.

The engines grumbled at each other as we sat at the end of the active runway awaiting instructions. When cleared for takeoff, I pushed the throttles full forward. The engines revved, noisy at the higher pitch, but smoothed out. I guided the plane along the centerline using small rudder adjustments. In the cold, dense air, we used little runway.

Once we were airborne, the Chugach Range filled the windshield.

Dale triggered the landing gear to retract. After the doors closed around the wheels, the climb improved, a little steeper and a little smoother. We gained altitude and I made gentle turns, first north and then westward, bringing the Alaska Range into view.

We left the Merrill Field control area and Dale did the radio work contacting Anchorage Approach Control to tell them our position and ask permission to cross their airspace. Once approved, he switched radios to tell Cecil our position and expected time en route.

With him handling all the communications, I could pay attention to flying.

At cruise altitude, Dale fine-tuned the fuel mixture, leaning it for improved fuel consumption and reduced engine wear. The engines grumbled during the changes, as if fighting with each other and then eased into a synchronous reassuring rumble.

We flew across Cook Inlet, over gray choppy seawater covered with dull chunks of ice carried in and out by tidal movement. Mount Susitna, a prominent landmark, drew closer. When we reached cruise altitude, Dale engaged the autopilot and locked the plane on course.

My eyes tracked a large ice block on the water. "It's nice to be at altitude with two engines holding us up over that cold water, isn't it?"

"Yeah. Down in Alabama where I grew up, if you went into the 'drink,' you'd probably survive if a gator didn't get you 'cause the water is warm. Up here, you're a goner in the cold water. You'd die of hypothermia." Dale adjusted the fuel mixture on both engines. "I like two engines. Just takes more concentration than a single."

"I'm not very alert after so little sleep. Would you take over? I think I'll just sit back and watch an expert. Thanks for letting me take off."

He showed me an exaggerated smile.

We reached the shoreline, bringing close the soft contours of Mount Susitna, the mountain resembling a sleeping woman. Behind Sleeping Lady lay a smaller mound, Little Mount Susitna. Dale broke my thoughts. "McGrath is about two hundred air miles from Anchorage. In the twin, it will only take us about an hour and a half. The most dangerous part of the flight is through Rainy Pass. I'll show you the route when we get there."

Initially the flight remained smooth, but after about thirty minutes, gusty headwinds swept out of the northwest, our direction of flight. The winds slowed our speed and buffeted the plane, but the autopilot held us on course. I focused on the GPS, which showed our route and ground speed. The time en route showed fifteen minutes longer than expected due to the headwind. This meant higher fuel consumption, but I knew we had enough.

The white featureless terrain below us provided few landmarks. To the north, the tops of Mount Denali and Mount Foraker pushed up, visible above the clouds blanketing their lower slopes. Clouds in our direction of flight loomed thicker and lower. The intimidating view made me tense. "Dale, I hate bad weather flying. It was nearly two by the time we took off. We'll be there long before dark, won't we?"

"Lots of time, girl. We're just coming up on Rainy Pass." Dale pointed to the terrain ahead. "Going west is not a problem. The mountains funnel us into the pass, so the route is obvious. Returning, the route is ambiguous, so I use a chant: *First left, first right, second left, second right*." The little mic situated to the left of his mouth carried his message to my ears. "Kelly, say that after me and commit it to memory. First left, first right, second left, second right."

I looked at him, wondering why he was emphasizing that.

"It's the directions through the pass. Eastbound, it zigzags, and you can't tell by the terrain what the real route is. Forget, and you'll find yourself in a blind canyon, slamming into a mountain." He looked at me to be sure I was paying attention. "There are crash sites everywhere out there."

I was on edge, wondering why I'd agreed to come.

Repeating the directions over and over provided distraction.

The cloud levels moved lower.

Dale cut the power and decreased our altitude, so he could fly beneath the cloud layer.

Soon we were flying around cloud stragglers hanging well below the overcast.

We flew around scattered snow showers. Occasionally, we'd fly right into one and lose visibility altogether. I finally asked. "Don't you think we should turn back? I'm getting nervous."

"It's not that fucking bad. Get ahold of yourself, girl," he snarled. "I've seen it worse than this. If you don't like my flying, you take over." He lifted his hands off the yoke.

"No. You fly this thing!" I took my hands off the yoke and scanned ahead to be sure he was keeping us below the clouds. "You know I don't like low visibility. I also don't like the lower altitude."

Dale gripped the controls. "We're exiting the pass now, so we're home free." A few minutes later, he glanced at the GPS. "I've had to dodge weather so much it has slowed us down and forced us to the south. We have plenty of fuel, but we're about 80 miles out from McGrath. It's to the north." He abruptly banked left and cut power to stay beneath the cloud layer. "We'll have to fly further south than I wanted to remain clear of clouds and snow flurries. If the weather pushes us lower still, I can stay under the clouds and turn north when we get to the river."

We'd be safer flying over a frozen river with no terrain to worry about.

Dealing with unknowns—such as by running into dense flurries, blizzard-like whiteouts, flying in clouds without radar or flight following, or being lost over the tundra with little likelihood of surviving a crash or of being found if we did survive—set my nerves on fire. I clenched my teeth to avoid exploding. I didn't find Dale's nonchalance reassuring.

"Be on the lookout for the Kuskokwim. I'll just follow its curves into town. We won't hit anything if we're right over the river." He laughed. "Based on our winds, we'll be landing to the north. Not to worry. When we get there, I'll buy you a beer at the Roadhouse to calm your frazzled nerves."

I tried to hide my rising anxiety with a faked smile. My dad had taught me to fly. We had flown in low-cloud conditions but always had an out—an alternate place to land, a turnaround plan, more than enough fuel. He didn't take chances, yet he died in a plane crash through no fault of his own. Another plane struck us midair on our final approach to the landing, destroying his ability to control the plane.

I had trusted Dad's skills, but this loss of control, being carried along by Dale with his willingness to take chances over unforgiving terrain, gripped my chest. My arms felt weak. I couldn't breathe.

We flew into snow showers. I could see nothing straight ahead; we were flying more than 200 mph into a whiteout. I expected a thud and sudden death.

Ominous.

I wanted sun and clear skies, but the skies had been clear when my dad and I had felt the sudden impact that sent our plane out of control.

I thought I'd recovered from that crash long ago, but my burn scars still haunted me, and now the scars burned and the rod in my leg felt cold. I wanted to run, but my seat belt held me firm. Death in the wilds of Alaska seemed as surreal as the stabbing in Seattle that had nearly taken my life. A panic attack surged. I wanted to grab the controls and climb, fly above the clouds, and head back to Anchorage, but we'd never make it—we would run out of fuel.

We had to go on to McGrath.

No way out.

No turnaround.

Take deep slow breaths.

Focus on the instruments.

Look for the river.

Talk to Dale.

Heavy snow showers blocked forward visibility for minutes that seemed to last forever.

Dale paid attention to the flying. We flew out of the snow.

He dodged clouds, sometimes too close to the ground.

We were losing daylight.

A snaky white line marked the land. I peered out my side window and tapped Dale's arm. "I see a river." The cloud layer thinned.

Dale lowered the right wing to look. I pointed to the frozen, serpentine river.

"Good eyes." He leveled the wings. "Thanks. That's the Kuskokwim."

Flying about three hundred feet above ground level, Dale followed the river's meandering course toward McGrath, where the river nearly encircled the runway in one sweeping loop. Runway lights guided us along the final course even though clouds still obscured the sun.

At three forty-five, it appeared much later due to the winter darkness setting in.

We crossed midfield and checked a wind sock parallel to the ground. That confirmed that we should land to the north. Dale turned and set up the downwind leg of our landing pattern. He called the Unicom radio repeatedly.

Someone finally answered. "Winds favor runway 34. Thirty-knot wind with gusts to thirty-six. No one else reported in the vicinity."

Dale announced, "CAP Cessna 310, Five Niner Six, turning left downwind. Landing runway 34, McGrath."

Gear doors opened. The plane shuddered as the gear locked down and the green wheels-down light flickered and then held steady.

We turned to final approach and touched down near the end of a plowed strip heading 340 degrees, nearly straight north.

A row of small planes sat huddled along the taxiway. Engines and wing covers protected, two taildraggers on skis were being buffeted by the wind. The only tricycle-gear plane other than the 310 we had just landed was a lone Cessna 172 parked near the fuel shack.

Snow berms stacked five feet tall by diligent snow-removal employees blocked our views to each side. I likened the berms to the sides of a luge; the embankments kept us on course. The plane slowed as Dale braked on the icy surface. He turned ninety degrees onto the taxiway to park along the east end of runway 7-25.

My anxiety had built to near combustion, although I had tried to act calm under the extreme duress and lack of control while flying with Dale.

Trapped.

Unable to get out.

Forced into bad weather. Flying dangerously low over obscured terrain. I feared they'd be searching for Dale and me, along with the lost musher, in the desolate, unforgiving wilderness.

The moment the gear touched down, I wanted to eject. As soon as the plane stopped, I opened the door and sucked in a deep breath of icy air. Clutching a small pack of essentials, I stepped out onto the wing. Nonskid tread and a handhold stabilized my route as I stepped down to the retractable step and then to the ground.

In my rush to get out of the damn plane, I slipped. My feet skidded on the icy ground, and I landed on my back. My parka blunted the impact.

Dale watched from his perch on the wing. "You'll have to go back to charm school. That isn't what I'd call graceful."

I struggled to my feet and watched him step off the wing, laughing. Then he hit the same slick spot I did and fell against me. I pushed him upright. "I hope no one saw this little show or we'll never live it down. We look like a couple of drunken sailors."

Dale laughed. "We will be as soon as we get to the Roadhouse." He pulled large wing covers from the baggage compartment. The wind caught them like parachutes. It took both of us to control and strap them to the wings. The activity distracted my anxiety.

"It's a pain to have to do this, but we won't have to de-ice the wings in the morning before the search." Dale fastened the last strap securing the nylon covers on the wings. "My hands are freezing. Let's get over and join the boys." He pointed to a large building.

From the air, the small collection of buildings called McGrath had looked abandoned. No neon lights. No vehicles. "I didn't see a motel when we flew in. Do they have rooms?"

"No. The town opens the high school gym. When I was here for a search last summer, we slept on the floor." Dale pulled his hood up and scanned the sky. "That's better than out in the brutal weather on the trail with Rollie. I hope he isn't injured."

"Maybe they'll have news at the Roadhouse." I was worried about the missing dogs, too.

We walked about a hundred feet to a two-story wood structure located between the end of the taxiway and the river. Loud music and laughter met us. "Sounds like we're late for a party." I tromped up the steps at the front of the building and waited for Dale to catch up.

He opened the door and stepped aside to let a staggering couple pass. "I've never been here when it wasn't party time. I owe you a beer to settle your nerves." We watched the couple stumble down the steps, heading along an empty street toward barking dogs. "Those CAP guys that arrived ahead of us are chicken-shit fliers to quit searching so early."

"Anybody would be crazy to fly in this weather," I muttered as we walked into the noisy bar. I doubted he heard my comment. A blast of warm air reeking of beer, cigarette smoke, onions, and grease engulfed us at the center of the universe of an Alaskan bush town with five hundred year-round residents.

From a table of six men, someone called to Dale. Close proximity to other tables made conversation easy. I recognized the faces of some CAP fliers from Anchorage. One man stood and pulled a chair in next to him. "This is for the lady. Dale, you'll have to find your own."

Dale placed a hand on my shoulder. "Guys, this is Dr. Kelly McKay. She works ER at Regional and flies with us on lots of CAP searches."

I pulled off my down jacket and hung it on the chair back.

Dale added, "I talked her into helping out on this search even though she'd worked all night."

I said hello and sat down.

"I scared the hell out of her flying here in this weather. The lady needs a drink."

Dale went to the packed bar located along a far wall. He returned with a pitcher of beer and glasses. He poured two and handed one to me. He signaled a barmaid. "I'd like a shot of whisky. You look like you need one, Kelly."

"No, thanks. I just need a beer, food, and sleep."

An older man beside me said, "I don't try to keep up with this crowd. One beer, then coffee for me."

"Good plan. We ate sausage and eggs at Peggy's about noon, but my stomach tells me it's time to eat."

"This is the only place in town, so you might as well order. Most of us are sleeping three blocks down the road at the high school." The man gestured in the direction the drunk couple had taken. "I'm turning in early. The search is on for tomorrow if we can see where we are going in this storm."

Men of all ages sat around the table. Dale found a chair and pulled it up at the far end. As he drank, Dale got louder and more vulgar. I counted him drinking three beers and three shots in less than the hour it took me to drink my beer and eat my burger. One of the guys asked him, "Why aren't you sitting by the lady? You'd better watch her with all the loose men around here."

"Kelly can take care of herself." Dale poured himself another beer. "I'm hooked up with her rich-broad roommate. She takes good care of me."

I hated his comments about Lynn. I shot him daggers and stood to leave. One of the guys said, "Kelly, it's time to party."

"I'm too tired. Maybe tomorrow night if we're still here."

"You know where to find us if you change your mind. We'll be back here at seven a.m. for a search briefing."

"I'll see you in the morning." I took my gear and walked in the icy air to clear my lungs of bar odors. Sudden wind gusts swirled snow, making it difficult to see. Flakes struck my face in icy jabs and collected on my lashes. A tail-wagging dog came down off a porch to greet me. Near the school, a dozen exhausted dogs tied to a fence sheltered from the wind curled up nose to tail. Snow stacked around the furry mounds, turning them into snowballs. They looked more tired than I did. They had run all the way here and I had flown, but I felt so tired I'd even sleep with the dogs.

A creaking door opened into an empty gym. Stashes of backpacks and sleeping bags belonging to bar patrons who were searchers lined the perimeter. I rolled out my thin foam mattress away from the door to avoid drafts and crawled into my sleeping bag fully dressed except for my boots. My rolled jacket made an acceptable pillow.

Periodically, whispered voices and snores awakened me until I stuffed foam plugs in my ears. Figures in sleeping bags lay at various angles on the hardwood floor. At 3 a.m., I searched the room for Dale but didn't see him. I changed position, covered my head, and fell back to sleep.

Chapter 5 McGrath, Alaska

An aching back and full bladder awakened me at five, feeling rested even though I'd awakened a few times from sleeping on the hard floor. I carried my sleeping bag and other belongings into the bathroom. Pipes rattled and produced an icy stream for brushing my teeth, splashing my face, and washing my underarms. Rough paper towels partially dried my skin.

A cold wind whipped my damp face and sent my teeth chattering. I suddenly felt very alone as I walked along the narrow, deserted street under a dark sky. I was a visitor in a foreign land, yet I didn't feel afraid.

Here, residents opened their homes to strangers and greeted people they didn't know like long-lost friends. Dale said most visitors only stayed long enough to refuel their planes. A few visitors came to fish at the convergence of the Takotna and Kuskokwim Rivers, but warmer days hatched swarms of mosquitoes and blood-hungry no-see-ums that drove people away.

Along my route, I glimpsed the dimly lit interiors of simple two- to four-room homes. Scattered streetlights cast shadows on yards where large mounds of pure white snow covered hidden treasures. VW Bug ghosts. Dead trucks. Wintertime transportation, snow machines and four-wheelers, were parked haphazardly near front doors.

The dog team I'd seen on my way to the school the preceding night was gone. Snow drifted into the dogs' impressions in the snow along the fence. White dust half-filled their tracks leading out of town back on the trail to Nome.

The smell of fresh coffee wafted out to greet me before I reached the Roadhouse. I left my gear in an alcove near the door and walked to a table of friendly guys hunched together eating eggs and hash browns. "May I join you?"

"Hi, Kelly. Please do." Smitty and I had met in Anchorage. He introduced me to the others.

I removed my jacket and hung it on a chair before wedging myself between two of the men. Bulky jackets hung on chair backs, providing a ring of colorful fabric beneath glaring lights. The thick warm air permeated with cooking smells and stale beer made me feel oxygen starved. "Any news on the lost musher?"

My acquaintance said, "No news. Those of us who didn't drink too late wanted to get an early start on the search. But the weather isn't cooperating. Forecast is for low visibility, blowing and drifting snow."

A bearded man in his sixties with an official Iditarod badge on his jacket walked over to our table. "I talked to Tom, our radioman at Cripple Creek, last evening. He had no word on the musher. Weather's awful out there." The man poured more coffee for himself from a carafe. "His Cessna 170 is drifted to the windows. Glad to be here and not out in a tent."

The official explained that some searchers had retraced trails by snow cat looking for evidence of where the lost musher might have taken a wrong turn, but they came back due to blizzard conditions. I looked at a map on the table. The man next to me pointed. "The mushers pass through here, head north to Cripple Creek, Ruby, and then turn westward to Galena. It's a tough area even when you can see where you're going."

After breakfast, we walked en masse to the refueling shack. A relentless north wind was blowing straight down the runway, and the windsock stood straight out. An occasional break in the fast-moving cloud layer gave us hope for better weather.

We huddled against the building out of the wind, watching a young man on a four-wheeler plow snow away from the parked planes. He blasted through drifts along the taxiway while a large truck with a snow blower disappeared in clouds of white as it cleared the runway.

A CAP pilot stomped his feet to stay warm. "I'm heading back to the Roadhouse. We can watch the weather from there. If it improves, they'll have the runway ready and some of us can begin the search." We followed him back along the route we had just taken.

The guy walking next to me scanned the sky. "If it clears a little, I'm going to go take a look-see. I've got my Super Cub on skis and will go by myself if no one wants to chance it."

Inside, warming my hands on another cup of coffee, I looked around. "Has anyone seen Dale? Maybe he's at the high school with a bad hangover."

"Dale? No. Dale was up to his usual. Drinking too much, too long, and enjoying the women. He left the bar with a local native honey about two."

I winced. The jerk. Drunk. Sleeping around. Lynn should know.

I hated to be the one to tell her.

Chapter 6 Alone in the Alaskan Bush

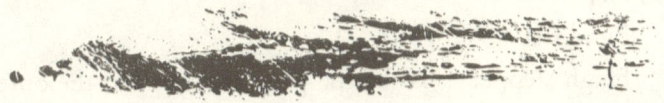

Dale still hadn't shown up at the Roadhouse by noon. The sky improved. At the search coordination meeting, local resident Hugh Denver, in his fifties, a part-Native seasoned Alaskan, invited me to fly with him. I accepted but had qualms about flying with someone I didn't know, and in an airplane that had seen better days.

However, a Super Cub on skis, only big enough for two people sitting one behind the other, sounded better than flying in a twin at low altitude with someone who'd been up drinking half the night. We could land almost anywhere on skis and survive, but that wasn't true of the large 310. Engine failure in a twin at low altitude gave the pilot little time to recover or stabilize the plane on the remaining engine before crashing.

Two aircraft engines cranked repeatedly, failing to start in the cold. Hugh and I climbed into his tandem two-place taildragger. I felt better when I saw the plane had dual controls. I could fly it from the back seat if necessary.

Hugh appeared to be a seasoned pilot, but the low cloud ceiling gave me second thoughts about agreeing to fly with him in such borderline weather. Hugh pushed the starter. The plane groaned. After five tries and nothing but groans from the engine, he announced, "The battery's almost dead.

The cold really gets to them. I should have taken it home and kept it in the house last night." He unfastened his seat harness. "Could you stand on the brakes while I get out and prop it?"

I nodded.

Hugh stepped close to the prop and gripped the outer quarter with heavy mitts. In a rapid movement, he dragged the tip downward and quickly stepped back to stay out of its way in case the engine started.

Nothing happened.

Hugh repeated the process. After numerous tries, the engine coughed and caught. In his bulky clothing, Hugh struggled back into the cockpit, smiling. He clamped the headset over his orange knit hat. "It'll be damn cold in the cockpit when we're flying. Super Cubs are leaky and noisy anyway, but my door is loose. It rattles from motor vibration." Hugh pulled the door shut and secured the latch. "Don't worry if it pops open in flight. It's no big deal to close it, but I might need you to grab the stick and fly while I'm doing it. I meant to get it fixed before winter hit but didn't get around to it."

I hoped there weren't other maintenance items he'd failed to fix.

Takeoff rolls on wheels from smooth pavement were much shorter than those from snow, rattling along on noisy skis. As lift increased with speed, the bumping sound decreased and the ride smoothed out.

Airborne.

Each search plane had a grid area assigned to it to reduce the likelihood of planes crashing into each other.

Hugh climbed beneath the cloud layer and altered our route after gaining enough altitude to clear terrain. "Our search grid is about fifty miles from McGrath, north of Cripple Creek. I've hunted there since I was a boy."

Cold air seeped in around the loose door. Hugh's voice crackled in my headset. "I'm keeping the heater and defroster blasting to warm it up in here a little and keep the windshield free of frost. I hate to use the heater much 'cause I got carbon-monoxided from it once. Gave me bad judgment."

That really made me feel confident.

I hoped he had had the heater fixed before this flight. A rattletrap airplane and a pilot with bad judgment. What had I gotten myself into?

Sun soon filtered through the thin cloud layer and cast a faint shadow of our airplane that followed us on the ground. The clouds dissipated, and this increased my comfort level. Hugh climbed higher. Once we reached our grid location, we flew a pattern of crisscrossing straight lines and sharp turns while scanning the ground for evidence of the musher and his dogs.

I kept an eye on Hugh's airspeed and watched the ground. Our pattern of low-altitude sharp turns increased the risk of losing lift, stalling the plane, and crashing. Maintaining proper airspeed on the sharp turns prevented stalls. Hugh paid attention to flying in gusty winds and irregular terrain. His airspeed never wavered. I appreciated his precision and, after assessing his skills, paid less attention to his flying and more attention to searching the ground.

By two o'clock, the wind stopped blowing us off course. Smoother air had less tendency to make me motion sick as my eyes scanned the dull winter landscape swept with gray shadows.

I looked for anything on the ground that might appear unnatural. I hoped Hugh's headset would work well enough to hear me above the engine and cockpit noise. "Do you know what color parka the lost musher wore?"

He nodded. "Red. I talked to him at the Roadhouse before he left for Nome. Nice guy from Minnesota named Rollie Erickson."

After twenty minutes of boring flying, I thought I saw something. "Turn back and look along the curve of that frozen creek."

Hugh put the plane into a sharp bank and turned 180 degrees. "Point out the spot."

I motioned. "Right down there where the creek hooks north. I see something moving along the bank."

"I don't see anything. Let's go down a little closer." Hugh reduced power.

I focused my binoculars. "It's a bunch of dogs. They're either tangled or tied to the trees along a steep bank."

Hugh turned again. "I thought at first it was a pack of wolves, but they didn't scatter. For sure, it's a string of dogs in harness yapping at us. Do you see a sled?"

"No."

Hugh circled again. "I'll make a low pass. Maybe I can land on a flat spot along the ridge across from the creek. The stream takes too many turns to land on it." Hugh flew low, examining the ridge. "Looks like a perfect landing spot."

I tried to make out more details regarding the dogs. At the top of the embankment, I saw something. "I think there's an overturned sled above the dogs."

"The ridge looks good. I don't see any rocks sticking up. Make sure your seat belt's tight." He chuckled. "You know, without brakes, you just hope to run out of speed before you run out of runway."

Dang. No brakes on skis.

I like wheeled planes with brakes, but we wouldn't be able to land here on wheels.

Hugh's voice crackled again. "I went lumberjacking right off into the woods one time. Broke off a couple of nice trees and took off a wing."

I smiled at his casual attitude, but an incident like that so far from help and on a rescue mission didn't appeal to me. I hung onto my seat belt and paid attention to his landing technique.

After a whisper touchdown, snow friction decelerated the small plane. Hugh kept the speed up enough to turn around and backtrack along our landing route. When we reached a wide enough area, he turned and repositioned the plane facing into the light wind, ready for takeoff.

Hugh reached behind my seat in the baggage compartment and brought out two pairs of round snowshoes. I carried a small backpack with chemical heat packs and a thermos of hot coffee to share if we found the musher alive. The snowshoes kept us from sinking into deep snow while we made our way to the other bank.

"Rollie!" Hugh yelled, "Rollie, are you up there?" The distressed dogs barked incessantly.

I stopped walking and listened. "I don't hear a response. He might not be able to hear you."

We set out along a gradual incline to the sled instead of trying to make it up the steep bank near the dogs. We made it to the level area above the creek near a collection of scrub pines, out of breath. We walked into a clearing and stared.

Ahead lay the broken, overturned sled and three blood-stained dead dogs, still in harness and connected to their distraught teammates. New snow covered some of the blood, but the drifts left gruesome stiff body parts exposed. The sled cover flapped in the wind. Fearing the worst, I stepped forward to look beneath the canvas.

Hugh trudged up behind me. "This doesn't look good."

Suddenly, a snarling dog burst from beneath the canvas.

I jumped back. "Good dog. It's okay. We won't hurt you."

The thin gray dog with blue-white eyes bared his teeth.

"Whoa, boy, whoa. Good dog," Hugh said as he stumbled backward to get away.

"Good dog." I called, "Anybody home in there?"

A growl from the on-guard young dog showed perfect white teeth. Paw prints and impressions from where he'd been lying packed the snow along the sled.

A startled voice from beneath the sled cover rang out. "Blue Boy, what is it?"

The dog wagged his tail and looked at the sled. The tarp lifted.

Hugh walked closer. "Rollie, you all right?"

"I'm hearing voices! Blue Boy, come here. It's okay."

Blue Boy sat near the sled. I squatted down and talked to the dog.

The dog's lips parted. A growl started deep in his throat. "Blue, it's okay." The musher dragged himself partway out of the shelter, grimacing with each movement. He held the dog's collar. "Blue won't hurt you if I tell him not to."

I pushed back my hood. "What happened?"

"Met up with a moose." Rollie crawled out farther. "Thanks for finding me. I took a wrong turn in a whiteout and kept going, thinking the trail was out there somewhere." He moved away from the sled, scooting on his butt because of a leg injury. "We were on the creek for a while, and then I followed what looked like the remnants of the trail when we ran up on a bull moose."

That would explain the dead dogs.

"We scared him. He charged and stomped the dogs, then got his leg tangled in the dog line." Rollie looked at his dead dogs and shook his head. "He dragged us through the trees a short distance before he freed himself and ran off." Rollie gripped his leg. "My leg got caught between the sled and a tree. Snapped. Broke halfway between the knee and ankle."

"You're in luck, Rollie." Hugh motioned to me. "This is Kelly McKay. She's an ER doctor from Anchorage."

"Thanks for being here." He patted his injured leg. "It's a half-assed job. I splinted it with a hatchet and duct tape. Grinds and hurts like hell when I move. I broke a few ribs, too. We've been here two nights."

Hugh squatted beside Rollie. "So sorry, but you're alive. We all were worried about you. The weather was too bad to search until today."

I pulled out the thermos. "How about some hot coffee?"

"God, that sounds good." I poured a cup in the thermos cap and handed it to him. "Are you cold?" I dug in the pack for the chemical warmers.

"Nah. I'm warm. Been lying under the tarp with Blue. Lots of food. I couldn't get out to untangle the dogs, but I threw them food, so they're fine." He glanced at the dead dogs. "My three honeys that got trampled broke my heart. The moose killed two skilled lead dogs I'd raised from puppies. I cried more over them than my injuries or getting knocked out of the race. What do we do now?"

"There's only room for two in the plane. We could leave you here and come back by snowmobile. Or, I could leave Kelly here with the dogs, fly you out now, and come back later to get her and the dogs."

Rollie shook his head. "I wouldn't leave a lady out here all by herself."

"Don't worry about me. I love dogs, and I'm accustomed to snow. I grew up in Minnesota like you, Rollie. I'll stay."

"So, you're a hardy Minnesotan? That sounds good, if you're sure."

"You betcha." I laughed.

"Okay. Now I believe you. Only Minnesotans talk like that."

I sat on the snow beside Rollie. "Let me take a look at your leg, and then we'll tend to the dogs."

Hugh looked at the fading sun. "We need to get going if I'm going to get back to McGrath in daylight." He looked worried. "Kelly, are you sure you feel okay about staying here in the wilds by yourself?"

"I won't be alone. The dogs are here."

"I'll leave you my gun. It's in the bag attached to the sled handle."

"I always carry one when I'm flying." I patted my right hip. "I grew up flying and shooting with my dad."

"No kidding. I'm from Hibbing, up on the Iron Range."

"I grew up in Cass Lake, just down the road."

"Okay, you two. No more socializing," Hugh cut in. "Kelly here is a doctor, so she knows what to do with that leg of yours. Let her at it."

"Man, how could I be so lucky as to be rescued by a pretty lady who's a doctor and almost from my hometown?"

Rollie gritted his teeth, held his injured leg and dragged himself to a tree to lean against it. Blue stuck to his side.

"Nice job on the splint. Isn't duct tape wonderful?" Rollie had placed the blade parallel to his foot and wrapped a hatchet along the outside of his injured leg with duct tape. "No survival pack is complete without duct tape. Can you wiggle your toes?"

He nodded.

"Can you feel your toes?"

"They are cold, but I have feeling. I kept checking on that. I think my foot is fine."

"You have such a good splint on, I think it's best if we just leave it in place since the feeling and circulation are good. I'll put an extension on it to stop the knee from bending. It will move less and not hurt as much."

I looked around for a splint. "It looks like one sled runner is history. Okay if I take a piece of it to lengthen your splint?"

"Sure. It will make a keepsake for the wall when I get home. I'll have people sign my runner instead of my cast." He smiled. "Don't know how I can thank you both enough." His voice dropped. "I was wondering if I could take Blue with me. We haven't spent a night apart since he was born. We really depend on each other."

"Not a problem. Let's go to the plane so we can get airborne. McGrath is about an hour flight time. Kelly, are you sure about staying out here overnight?"

"That's fine if you don't forget where I am. I'd much rather be here than working in the ER. Take your time."

"I have the GPS coordinates, so I know exactly where to find you. We'll return by snowmobile if the weather closes in."

Rollie slid down the slope on his butt as I supported his leg. Once on the frozen creek, he placed his arms over our shoulders and hobbled between us. Soon we had him wedged into the back seat with his splinted leg resting between the pilot's seat and the door. The battery had charged during our flight, and the engine started on the first try. Blue curled up on Rollie's lap and didn't even lift his head when the prop caught. The plane sped away from me along the frozen ridgeline, leaving in a cloud of prop-blasted snow. After the air cleared, I watched the small plane climb above the trees and turn toward McGrath. After a wing wave, they disappeared from view over the scrub pines.

Alone in the wilds of Alaska.

I wondered when they'd return but didn't really care.

No anxiety. No people. No rush. No one trying to die and no one trying to kill someone.

Peace. Total peace.

We had found the musher and his dogs. Now he could rest, too.

I trudged back to the sled.

The dogs whimpered. I sat down to drink the rest of my coffee and rested for a few minutes. I talked to the dogs and contemplated my tasks.

The wind came to visit. First it was a low whistle, and then moans rocked the treetops and dumped clumps of snow down around me from laden branches. Then the wind subsided, leaving me with the sound of dogs breathing, my own breathing, and my heart pounding from the uphill walk wearing snowshoes.

I dug around inside the sled and found bags of human and dog food, a large pot, a small camp stove with fuel, and a stash of Snickers. Stacks of frozen pan-size pizzas looked inviting. I helped myself to a candy bar and started to work, moving the dead dogs away from our camp area.

Using their harnesses, I dragged each carcass into the woods. The unbending limbs proved a challenge, but I removed the harnesses and later stashed them in a canvas bag I found in the sled. Then I moved each of the eight remaining dogs and tied them to individual trees surrounding the sled. They howled and did happy dances when I pulled out bowls.

Melting snow for water over the single-flame stove took a while, but soon the dogs happily lapped warm water and chomped down their food. It was probably not quite the process Rollie used but feeding that many dogs at once was a first for me. I petted each one and then surveyed Rollie's supplies.

After melting snow for dog water, I placed chocolate powder in my thermos with the remaining coffee and added boiling water. Cramping feet forced me to remove my boots. A wind sent chills up my spine, so I zipped my jacket and crawled into Rollie's sleeping bag. A tall black male dog with four white feet watched me with golden eyes.

I slid my boots on and walked over to unfasten his rope. He followed me to the sled and lay beside me. I examined his feet, not looking for sores, just curious. When weight-bearing, his toes splayed. He had big feet with webbed toes, his personal snowshoes. He watched me shyly and licked my hand. His fluffy black tail with a white tip thumped a couple of tired beats. His dark coloration, wide brow, and unusual golden eyes reminded me of a friendly black bear. I named him Boots.

I crawled into the sleeping bag. The dog moved closer and curled up against me as if he'd done it before. We lay together beneath the edge of the tarp in our own little den. I slept with my arm over his back.

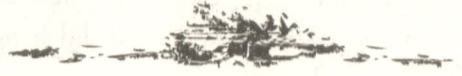

I awakened to blackness and disorientation. Elusive dreams had left me breathless. My sweet bed partner had left. I lifted the tarp. Sparse trees to the west provided a view of the star-sprinkled sky. I wiggled out of the sleeping bag and stood. Something bumped my leg, a nudge. "Boots, is that you?" I patted his head. "What should we do? I suppose you and the other dogs are hungry."

It was so dark.

I felt around under the tarp for a flashlight.

Nothing.

I rummaged in the bag attached to the rear handle of the sled, where I found more candy, nuts, and something furry. I pulled out Rollie's cap with fur earflaps and an attached headlamp. The bright beam flashed into a dark stand of trees. I scanned the area. Dogs stared into the beam with glowing eyes. I put the warm lighted hat on my head and let the earflaps blow in a light wind as Boots and I walked along to the edge of the bluff. The storm had blown through, leaving the sky totally clear.

Northern lights undulated across the sky in brilliant curtains of eerie green. Turning reddish, they flipped and crackled with the sound of static electricity. The stars appeared closer than I had ever seen them.

Overwhelmed by the intensity and beauty, I flipped off the headlamp and sat down to watch. Sheets of color, like ever-changing flames, waved and flickered overhead. I put my arm around the dog. "Boots, this is so beautiful. Is this what it's like to be a sled dog in the Alaskan wilderness? You're a lucky dog." I couldn't see his expression. He was probably thinking, *Yeah, stuck out here with a city girl. At least she knows how to fix dog food, and I can tell she likes me. Maybe she'll give me extra treats.*

"We slept a long time. We were all tired." My watch told me the time, 10 p.m. "I don't want to leave this view, but it's time to eat. After not eating much for days, I bet you're all hungry."

Desolate terrain surrounded me, yet I felt no fear.

The terrors of Seattle were erased.

My former life was nonexistent.

I found peace with eight dogs, miles from nowhere.

The headlamp provided focused light while giving me free hands to prepare each of the dogs a warm meal. After I fed and watered them, I turned to my own dinner and devoured a small pizza after heating it in a pan over the little stove. I topped it off with hot chocolate and a Snickers bar.

About midnight, Boots and I visited each dog. I petted them, and he exchanged friendly greetings of nose touching and sniffing. Then, we curled up together and fell asleep.

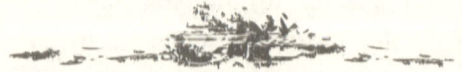

I awakened to the chaos of barking dogs. Boots tore from beneath the tarp, snarling. The other dogs emitted sharp barks and snarls. I jerked Rollie's hat onto my head, turned on the lamp, and pulled my 9-millimeter from its holster.

Boots pressed against my legs, staying between me and a circle of eyes.

Not dogs.

Wolves, a pack of wolves.

Boots lunged repeatedly but didn't leave my side.

Devil eyes flashed. Then, the thin gray figures disappeared, followed by a sudden ruckus of snarling and snapping from the area where I had stacked the dead dogs. The starving pack fought over the find and dragged the carcasses farther away to feast.

Rollie's dogs barked hysterically and wailed for at least an hour. When they finally quieted down, I crawled back beneath the sled flap, protected by the sled from behind and by Boots in front. His tense on-guard body remained within my reach. I felt chilled, trembling from the adrenaline surge, and was wide awake. I listened and waited for morning.

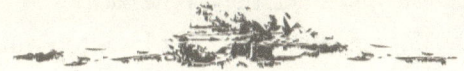

At sunup, the sound of a motor alerted me. Boots barked a sharp warning. The other dogs yipped. Some sounded like they were talking; others howled. I walked to the embankment with Boots and scanned the sky. The engine sound faded and then grew louder as a Super Cub set up to land.

Two men exited the plane and scrambled across the creek and up the embankment. The man who flew in with Hugh carried a sled runner. "Hi, Kelly. I've been hearing about you on the way out. I'm Joe Noyes.

Hugh greeted me. "Joe used to run a trap line and is a dog handler. He came out to help get the dogs back to McGrath."

Joe surveyed the dogs. "Are any of them hurt?"

"None of them appear injured. The marauding moose killed three. There are eight of them left."

Hugh asked, "Did you get cold last night?" I told them about sleeping beneath the protective tarp. "Boots kept me warm, and I slept for hours. I saw an awesome show of the northern lights. It was the most memorable night of my life. You could sell tickets to this place."

"Hugh, is this girl for real? By herself in the bush and happy?"

I laughed. "I loved it!" Then I told the men about the wolves.

Hugh tensed. "I knew we shouldn't have left you." He looked around the camp. "Are you really okay? That could have been catastrophic. Did they come back?"

"No. The dogs quieted down, but I was too wound up to sleep. This big guy protected me." I patted Boots. "I'm glad to see you."

Joe walked over to check the dogs. He scratched their ears, patted along their backs, and checked their feet and legs. Each of the cooperative dogs greeted him with barks and wags. "How do you like the dogs, Kelly?" Joe asked.

"They're great. I melted snow for water and fed them twice yesterday. I haven't fed them this morning." I pulled back the tarp to show him the food stash. "Be sure to find Rollie's pizzas. They're good. He also has a stash of candy bars. That's all I needed."

"I'm sure I'll find some good stuff. He had enough to get him to Nome." Joe picked up the stove. "There's a team of three snow machines en route carrying a GPS and radios, all towing sleds. No one will get lost this time."

"Are you going to run the dogs?" I gazed longingly at the dog team and hugged Boots.

"The dogs look fine. If I get Rollie's sled functional with the new runner, I'll run the dogs to McGrath along the snow machine trail."

The two men offloaded some of Rollie's gear and turned the sled over. Hugh trudged back to the plane to get tools to help remove broken pieces. After more than an hour of figuring out how to secure the runner so it would hold for the long trip, Joe felt sure their plan would work.

"I'll feed the dogs after you two take off." Joe admired their sled repair.

I petted a friendly blue-eyed dog. "I wish I could go back by ground with you."

Hugh shook his head. "Dale asked when I would have you back after I told him last night you stayed here with the dogs. He said he was going to the Roadhouse to hang one on and fly back today."

"That sounds like Dale, drinking too much. Guess I'd better get back to McGrath to go with him."

Joe nodded. "It could be a tough ground trip. The snow is deep in places and will be slow going. It could take us ten hours."

Hugh tightened a strap on one of his snowshoes. "We better head back. It may already be too late for you to return to Anchorage. There was more weather coming in."

"You better get going." Joe looked at the sky. "Weather here looks okay."

"Did you bring a lantern, Joe?" Hugh wondered.

"No, but I'm sure Rollie has one."

"I found Rollie's headlamp." I removed the hat with attached headlamp straps and handed it to Joe. He put it on and waved us off. "Get goin'. Me 'n' the dogs'll be fine."

I didn't want to leave. I'd rather take my chances in a blizzard with a team of dogs and unknown men than face flying with Dale again.

Chapter 7 More Bad Behavior

On the way back to McGrath, Hugh invited me to stay overnight with him and his wife. "Suzie said to invite you for dinner. She's making moose stew and homemade bread."

"That sounds delicious. I'm starving."

"Suzie made up the roll-away in the back room for you. It'll be more comfortable than the gym floor."

"That would be great."

Hugh touched down near the end of the runway. The plane slowed rapidly. He added power and back taxied to the far end of the runway and turned onto the taxiway for parking. My unfounded worries about skidding off the runway due to no brakes had evaporated after landing on skis a couple of times. The friction of the skis on the snow slowed the plane rapidly, and he had to add power to reach his parking location. Hugh tied the plane securely in its designated spot. I helped him attach wing and engine covers to protect the fabric-covered airplane from the harsh weather and ice. Since it was March, daylight hours had increased, but by the time we landed, streetlights glowed against the darkening sky.

Raucous voices increased as we approached the Roadhouse on foot. A table of Hugh's friends called, "Congratulations! Have a beer on us."

We sat down. I really wanted food, not a beer. "Beer sounds good, but one beer will probably go right to my head," I said with a laugh.

"It's okay, Kelly, you deserve one. I'll carry you home if I have to, and Suzie will fill your stomach. You'll sleep better tonight. I promise, no wolves."

Hugh told them the wolf story. "Kelly is now a real Alaskan."

One of the men handed us each a beer and cheered.

Good beer and the camaraderie of friends today who were strangers yesterday made me feel as though I belonged. Alaskans fought the elements together and supported each other. I answered a few questions about the wolf encounter before asking about Rollie.

"He flew out with a film crew. They offered him a lift to Anchorage and wanted to interview him for a good story. It worked out great for everyone."

"What about his dogs?"

"He wanted to take Blue but wasn't sure what he'd do with him at the hospital. The old musher Ed Jensen, in Wasilla, is going to board all of them. After the snow machine brigade and Joe Noyes get them back here, we have volunteers who will fly them to the airport in Palmer not far from Ed's house."

"I know Ed and Lucille. It's nice of them to take in the dogs."

"I think everybody knows them." Hugh explained, "Rollie came up early to train his dogs for the race at Ed's. I imagine Rollie'll stay there after they fix his leg till he can travel back home."

I finished my beer.

"If we don't get home soon, Suzie will be here looking for me. She worries too much."

We said our goodbyes, picked up our gear, and left. I forgot to ask anyone about Dale but planned to return in the early morning, ready to leave for home.

Hugh pointed out a few old buildings and gave me some town history on the three-block walk to his home. We entered a comfortable living room warmed by a potbelly cast iron stove with a steaming copper kettle on top. Flames flickered behind a scorched pane in the door. Two overstuffed couches lined the walls, and delicious smells wafted from the kitchen. A beautiful Native woman with shiny black hair that hung to her waist appeared in the doorway.

Hugh squeezed his wife. "Hope we didn't keep you waiting too long."

Suzie greeted him with a gleaming smile.

"We had to drink one celebratory beer with the guys. Kelly could sure use some of your moose stew. Meet Kelly."

"Hi, Kelly. Come on in. I just took bread out of the oven. Dinner is almost ready."

"Dr. Kelly helped find Rollie and, like I told you, she stayed to care for his dogs till I could get back and pick her up today."

"I hope things went well. I wouldn't want to be out there alone." Suzie wore a crimson jogging outfit, no makeup, and was a striking beauty. "Are you a vet?"

"No, an ER doctor. I volunteer with the CAP and had a few days off so came out to search."

"Thanks for helping. Are you hungry?"

"Starving."

"Good." Suzie's cheery expression turned to a frown. "There'll be hell to pay over those dead dogs." She explained, "There are always investigations when a dog is ill or injured during the race. Animal cruelty people watch everything we do and want to ban the Iditarod."

"Anyone knowledgeable about the race and Alaska understands the moose danger. We're invading their territory, so there are problems once in a while."

I removed my jacket and sat on the arm of the couch as we talked. "It could have been worse. I'm glad Rollie survived."

Hugh hung our coats on wall hooks near the door. "Right. Dog deaths along the trail are not common. Vets are stationed at every checkpoint."

Suzie invited us to sit at a kitchen table covered with a red and white checkered cloth. "We drink powdered milk out here, Kelly. Air freight costs are too high to bring milk in by the gallon."

Hugh served each of us from a large pot. "I got this moose last fall. The meat will last us till next year." Hugh smiled. "Try the tundra milk, you may like it."

She poured milk for each of us from a large pitcher and sliced the bread. I ate till I was stuffed and decided I actually liked the powdered milk. I retired to my cot in the back room after washing up and brushing my teeth. I was too tired to socialize.

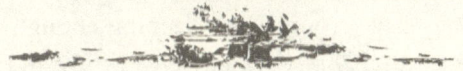

Suzie knocked on my door in the morning. "Coffee's on."

I rolled out of bed to the smell of coffee and toast. I appeared in the kitchen with bed hair and a sleep-creased face, wearing the same clothes I'd worn for three days. "You look like you could use this." Suzie met me with a cup of coffee. "I put out towels for you, if you'd like to take a shower."

I carried the coffee with me and in record time emerged after showering, brushing my teeth, and taming my damp hair in a ponytail of corkscrew copper curls. "Hope I didn't scare you when I walked out for coffee without combing my hair. It's so curly when it gets out of a clip or rubber band it's like a lion's mane. Sure wish I had beautiful hair like yours."

"Thanks, but I've always wanted curly hair. Women are never satisfied." Suzie smiled.

"This has been an interesting trip for me. Hugh is a very good pilot. He tells me you worry about him."

"I worry because he flies too much, ferrying people into the bush for hunting and fishing. During the summer, he's gone somewhere almost every day."

"Is he still sleeping?"

"Oh, heavens, no. He left hours ago. Went to the checkpoint down the street to see if Rollie's dogs got back. He came back about eight thinking you'd be up. It's ten now. I guess that means you slept well."

"It's unusual for me to sleep this late. I love mornings so usually get up early."

"You may have trouble not sleeping enough in Alaska summers. Morning comes about two a.m. around here. The sun barely goes down."

"You're right. When I arrived last summer, people told me to tape tinfoil to my bedroom window to keep the sun out. I didn't want to but gave in, and now I sleep better."

"Do you want some oatmeal and toast before you go find Dale? I have it all ready."

"Thanks." I ate while we talked. "Do you think Rollie will run the race again?"

"I'm sure he will. It gets in their blood. He got all the way to Nome last year, just not in the money."

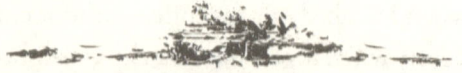

Suzie directed me to the McGrath checkpoint near the high school. I found a line of very tired dogs strung out and being patted, fed, and watered. Blue Boy sat forlorn at the end of the line. He wagged his tail when I walked up and hugged him. I hoped I'd see him again at Ed's. Hugh motored up on a snow machine.

"Good morning. I slept like a log. Suzie finally woke me. Are Rollie's dogs here yet?"

"We got a radio report. They're just a few miles out."

"Have you seen Dale?"

"I just left him at parking. Told him I'd give you a ride down to the 310. He's ready to roll."

The snow machine rattled and snorted like an idling chainsaw. My muscles complained when I climbed on, but I enjoyed an exhilarating ride through town and out to the airstrip.

We found Dale leaning against the fuel shack with his head buried in the hood of his parka. His hands were in his pockets, and he wasn't moving.

The line boy pulled up near him on a four-wheeler and slid to a stop.

Dale didn't look up.

Hugh stopped and left the snow machine running while I got off. "Thanks for the lift, great food, and the hospitality."

"Come back soon. You better go wake up Dale. He doesn't look too good, Doc." Hugh gunned the motor and headed to the Roadhouse.

Dale looked up. "Glad you could make it. I've been out here freezing my ass waiting."

One look at his face and I wondered if he should be flying. "Headache, Dale? How much did you drink last night?" Bloodshot eyes glared. "You're supposed to take two aspirin at night and call your doctor in the morning. Your doctor is here, but I don't have any aspirin. Looks like you could use some right now."

The line boy joined us. "Hey, Dale, Dad said you and Lulu were really knocking 'em down last night."

I laughed, but my gut clenched at the thought of him with another woman. "No wonder your head hurts. Want me to do most of the flying today? I got a good night's sleep at Hugh and Suzie's."

"Heck, no. I'm in perfect shape." He flipped back his hood and snarled, "I want you to do the flying when it's really shitty like it was when we flew in." Dale walked off toward the plane. Over his shoulder, he added, "Just kidding." He cleared his throat and spit into the snow.

He was an all-around gross individual. I hoped Lynn would dump him.

A large round thermometer on the outside of the fuel shack read minus 8. Just a whisper of icy wind blew out of the north, fluttering the wind sock and rotating it with a metallic screech.

We taxied to the end of the runway and took off into a cloudless sky.

Dale let go of the controls as soon as the wheels came up. "It's all yours. I'll lean it out and synchronize the engines when we reach seven thousand feet, then I'm going to snooze." He turned toward me, exhaling fumes of stale coffee and booze—mostly booze. "Don't say anything about Lulu to Lynn, okay?"

I looked at him in shock, "Dale, what the hell! Have you been drinking this morning?"

"I quit at midnight. Don't believe what the kid said. I'm good. I can fly drunk better than most pilots can fly sober. Besides, you're flying."

"I don't have a twin rating."

"You don't need one with me here. I'm pilot in command."

I looked straight ahead, holding the plane steady and climbing to the altitude he suggested.

Dale gripped my left arm and squeezed. "You heard what I said."

I jerked my arm from his tight grasp and sent the plane into a sharp bank to the left. He held on tight as I corrected and leveled the wings.

"Lay off, bitch. If Lynn finds out about Lulu, I'll know who told her."

Dale leaned back and closed his eyes. I shook him awake a few minutes later when we reached cruising altitude. He adjusted the engines, looking at instruments through half-lidded eyes. He folded his hands in his lap and closed his eyes. Clouds of whiskey-tainted air filled the cockpit.

I set the GPS for Anchorage but flew through Rainy Pass, repeating the route in my head like a song. Rugged mountain peaks at this altitude were easy to avoid when flying in clear skies, but I saw how pilots could get screwed up and become lost in bad weather. I wondered how Dale and I actually made it through on our way to McGrath with such poor visibility.

When we neared Anchorage, I radioed for clearance to transit the International Airport control space. I looked down on rivulets of receding tide painting corduroy waves in the sand on the shoreline of Cook Inlet. Approach Control came back with our clearance, Dale's breathing changed. He sat up straight and opened his eyes. He gazed down at the water and off at Anchorage in the distance.

"Looks like you found your way home." He dropped the gear and took the controls. "It's my airplane." He contacted Merrill Tower for landing.

Perfect landing. Dale was an excellent pilot, both helicopter and fixed wing, but I didn't respect him as a human being.

He dropped me off at the apartment and drove off without speaking.

Chapter 8 Fly by Night

Lynn's clothes still lay in a heap by the door. Dirty dishes were stacked in the sink. I changed into a pair of clean jeans and a turtleneck sweater and then threw a load of clothes in the wash and cleaned the house while wondering what to do or say about Dale's behavior. If he gave her a sexually transmitted disease after his escapades in McGrath, she'd kill him.

I didn't have to say anything. She knew some STDs are fatal. Was I saving our friendship, or was their relationship worth risking a dread disease and death? No. I just had to figure out when and how to tell her.

I called Ed and Lucille, and Lucille answered. "Hi, Dr. Kelly, Ed's out feeding the dogs. We hoped you'd call."

"I just got back from the search for your friend Rollie."

"We know. He called us from the hospital and told us you found him with Hugh. What a great coincidence that you're both from Minnesota."

"Are his dogs there yet?"

"The first arrived this morning. When are you coming out?"

"I have to work the next three-day shifts, then I have two days off before I go back to nights again. I could come out this weekend."

"Come for dinner Saturday and stay overnight. They are putting plates and screws in Rollie's leg this morning. He'll stay with us for a couple weeks when he gets out."

I hung up happy, looking forward to the weekend. I felt rested enough to do a little reading and Boards review. Lynn and I would be going back to Seattle to take the test in a couple months.

I dreaded being back in that city.

Lynn and Dale walked in about 7:30 p.m. He'd picked her up at the hospital after work. She was still wearing her scrubs. "Come on, Kelly, grab a jacket. I'm taking you girls to the Fly By Night Club for a drink and some of their delicious Spam hors d'oeuvres. Mr. Whitekeys is playing tonight."

Going anywhere with Dale was the last thing I wanted to do. Maybe he was trying to make up and keep things happy. I looked at Lynn, who said, "I haven't been there since last fall. It's a fun place. Let's go. You both need to lighten up. That trip to the bush must have been rough."

"Mr. Whitekeys' piano playing and the comedy skits with local references bring a packed house. We don't even serve Spam in Alabama." Dale laughed as we followed him out the door.

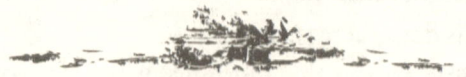

Once the piano music started and the songs began, the bar patrons howled with laughter at the songs. They munched peanuts, tossed shells on the floor, guzzled beer, and helped themselves to Spam tidbits. We laughed along with them. Dale slipped his arm around Lynn's shoulder and sipped his drink.

On a bathroom break, I told her I'd studied for the Boards.

"Good for you. My heart's not in it. Work is okay, but I'm tired of books."

"That's the way I feel, too, but it's only weeks away. I studied more last fall, when I was recovering, than I have in the past two months."

Lynn climbed back up on her highchair by Dale. There was only one choice of seating when we walked into the packed nightclub, but it provided a perfect view of the place. "Kelly and I have to fly to Seattle in April for our ER Board exams. I got my registration confirmation yesterday, Kelly. Yours didn't come."

"I looked through all the mail and didn't see anything from the Board. I hope there's no screw-up."

Lynn sipped the last of her beer. "It will be good to have the test over with."

"I'm as ready to take the exam as I'll ever be, but I dread going back to Seattle. Too many bad memories."

"You have to forget about your troubles. Speaking of trouble, I wonder how Brett Warren is?"

"I don't want to know."

Dale leaned closer. "So, Kelly, who's Brett?"

"Her ex-lover, ex-surgeon, a drug addict she left behind in Seattle. He was carrying on with other women behind her back and shooting up drugs."

"He's a psychopathic liar and a pretty boy." I took a slug of beer, angry that Lynn would even say his name. "If I never see him again, I'd be happy."

Dale looked down and said nothing. I wondered if his behavior was related to Lynn's tone about Brett's behavior with other women.

Back at our apartment, Dale dropped us off on the street. "Goodnight, ladies. I'm beat up after all that searching. I have to sleep. I'm on flight duty at zero seven hundred."

Lynn kissed him. "I don't work tomorrow. Sleep well, sweetie." She closed the car door.

"Thanks for the evening out. I'm on days, too." I waved and stepped back.

Dale drove off.

Lynn tossed her jacked on the couch. "I think Dale works way too many hours. I wish he'd take better care of himself."

After spending time with Dale and watching his behavior, I had to agree with her. Taking better care of himself should include less alcohol.

Chapter 9 Mushing

He's baaack. John asked especially for you." One of the nurses handed me a chart.

I read the name and stopped short.

"Don't worry. He's making sense, and this time he just has a couple of minor cuts."

John Reilly smiled from the end of a bed in the suture room. His curly black hair was combed. A long-sleeved red turtleneck covered his feather tattoos. Other than a few smears of blood on his jeans, he looked clean, normal, and strikingly good looking, like I remembered him from CAP flights.

"Dr. McKay, I hate to bother you with something minor. I slipped and cut myself using my pocketknife. I was whittling a bird to give you. I know you like big traumas like doctors on TV. This won't take you long, then you can get back to real doctor work."

"I'm surprised to see you out of the hospital already. How are you doing?"

"I was a very good boy. They turned me loose two days ago. I'm on Risperdal again. Down at CAP, they said you'd been out to McGrath with the rest of the boys and found the musher yourself. Those guys think you're great."

I dreaded talking with him about CAP and flying. Not allowing him to fly on searches might trigger a violent confrontation since flying meant so much to him. If he didn't report the violent episode, I would have to. Patient confidentiality regarding medical issues made the situation complex. I didn't want to encourage him by talking about CAP. "Are you hurt anywhere else?"

"No, just the cuts."

An RN prepared the suture tray, cleansing solutions, and sterile gloves for me. "Let me know if you need anything else here. Just yell." She left the room.

Birdman didn't flinch when I injected the local anesthetic into the laceration on his left hand. I sat close to his side as I worked and felt his eyes focused on my face. A perfect gentleman. As I was finishing, he leaned forward, looking at my hair. "You an Irish girl with all those red curls?"

I nodded.

"I'm Irish like you, Dr. McKay. You treat me nice. Will you take my stitches out when I come back?"

I told him I would.

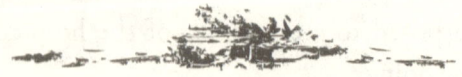

Lucille answered when I called them on Saturday morning. "Kelly, come right out. I have trapper stew on the stove for lunch and bread in the oven. A reporter will be here to interview Rollie about the moose incident."

I tossed my sleeping bag and a change of clothes in the back of my secondhand Subaru and headed out of town thinking about the Boards. The accumulated stack of mail contained no confirmation of my registration and payment to take the exam, which was just weeks away. Lynn had received hers, and we had our flight reservations.

A medical review tape on drug toxicity and overdose treatment kept me company en route from Anchorage, past the nice small town of Eagle River and along the beautiful scenery of Knik Arm, an extension of the Bay of Alaska. About the time the tape finished, I drove into Ed and Lucille's winding driveway where their white modular home sat on a small hill surrounded by scrub forest facing westward. The circle drive looked like a parking lot.

Barking dogs announced my arrival.

Lucille waved from the porch as I got out of the car. Dressed in red tights and a long pale blue sweatshirt, from a distance she looked like a teenager. Red combs behind each ear held her poufy hair back. Flour powdered the front of her sweatshirt, which was emblazoned with *Alaska, Where Men Are Men and Women Win the Iditarod*. She pulled me into an open living area with a combined living room, dining room, and kitchen that took up half of the house.

Cooking smells filled the air. Ed appeared ten years younger than the last time I had seen him. She poured me a cup of coffee, and Ed jumped to his feet to pull out a chair next to his. Not much taller than I, with his arm around my shoulders, he announced, "This is my doctor, Kelly McKay."

I smiled. Rollie waved from the couch where he lay with his leg up. Blue Boy curled on the couch with him. Al, their helper, was also there. A young woman with a press badge sitting at the table with Ed said, "Hi, Kelly. Ed and Rollie have been talking about how much you helped both of them."

Rollie called, "I'd get up and shake your hand, but my leg's broke." He laughed. "Thanks for saving my butt and taking care of my dogs, Doc."

"You're welcome, Rollie. I wondered how your leg was doing, but what I really wanted to do was come out and hug one of your dogs I named Boots."

"Is he black with white feet and golden-brown eyes?"

I nodded. "He kept me safe and snuggled with me in your sleeping bag after Hugh flew you back to McGrath."

"He's a lover boy. Sleeps with me all the time." He patted Blue Boy, who lay on the couch with him. I have terrific sled dogs from Ed's lineage."

"Dr. Kelly, I want you to meet all of them. You'll see the same markings, eyes, and personality traits as in Rollie's dogs." Ed motioned to a small black dog near Rollie. "This is Jack" The short-haired dog jumped up on Ed's lap and looked lovingly into his face. "Jack, show Dr. Kelly where the candy is. Maybe he wants some butterscotch."

The dog hopped down and pawed a kitchen drawer.

Ed asked the dog, "What do you say?"

Jack woofed politely, but when Ed headed for the drawer, he couldn't control himself and went into a dog dance.

Ed held up one hand and then made a downward motion.

Jack dropped into a lying position, paws forward, head alert, eyes locked on Ed's face.

"Good boy."

Ed slowly opened the drawer and painstakingly peeled the wrapper from a piece of butterscotch candy.

The dog waited like a statute.

Ed held the candy out for the dog.

Jack curled his lips back and gently took the candy from his fingers.

"Dogs are easy to train. They want to learn. You need to give them the rules, follow them yourself, and pay them with treats and pats on the head." He hugged Jack. "Just like babies, they learn what they're taught. If you have a child or a dog that doesn't behave, it's the owner's fault."

Jack listened to every word until Ed said, "Okay, go see Rollie."

The dog curled up on the floor beside his friend.

The reporter asked all the men more questions about training dogs and about traits for lead dogs. She inquired about the strange little dog who looked nothing like the sled dogs.

Lucille served large bowls of steaming stew and sliced bread. "We went to town to buy groceries about two years ago and found him as an abandoned puppy, freezing in the parking lot. I tucked him inside my coat. He's been ours ever since."

The trapper stew contained chicken, beef, moose, and pork, along with vegetables from their homegrown supply. Simmering for hours blended the flavors and produced a hearty meal. Before everyone but Rollie went outside after lunch, Lucille pointed to chickens thawing on the countertop. "You're all invited for dinner."

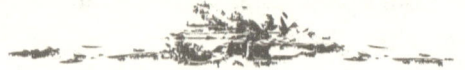

Rows of dog houses stretched for half a block along a snowmobile trail heading toward the forest. Dogs chained to stakes yipped happily. Many of them stood on top of their straw-stuffed box houses to get a better view of their visitors. Ed rapped the side of a shed three times with a large stick.

The dogs stopped barking. "It gets too loud out here with them all barking. I just teach them early on. I don't like them barking all the time. They sound a warning if a bear or moose comes near, so I like them to have the freedom to bark." He motioned to some dogs near us. "Rollie's dogs have boarded here before. They understand the no-barking rule."

Al and Ed harnessed up six dogs and hooked them three to a sled. After a few instructions, the reporter and I had our own teams mushing alone behind the men on a snow machine leading the way along a trail into the woods. Before we set out, I told Ed I worried about the dogs carrying my weight.

"Honey, you're a lightweight. We're running the snow machine ahead of you to slow down the teams. After you have more experience, I'll set you free."

The trail wound through gnarled pine woods with stunted growth to a small lake where we stopped to rest. Al shut down the snow machine. The woods turned silent but for the breathing of the dogs and an occasional stellar jay announcing our presence to other forest creatures.

I sat down on my sled, out of breath from pumping, helping the dogs, like we were taught to do in our two-minute lesson. "This is wonderful, Ed. In one ride, you have me hooked."

The reporter smiled brightly and dug out a camera secured around her neck beneath her parka. She took some photos. "This is the best assignment I've had in a long time. Thanks so much. You and Al sure know how to handle dogs."

Al, shy and quiet, said, "Ed taught me everything I know. He's a good teacher."

After the ride, we gathered at the table with Lucille for more coffee before the reporter reluctantly left on her drive back to Anchorage. The evening passed quickly with comfortable conversation, chicken dinner, more bread, a little television, and two hours of playing Uno.

Rollie slept on the couch with Blue. I slept on another couch in the living room, snuggled in my sleeping bag. In the dark, Rollie and I talked about Minnesota till I heard his breathing slow. I closed my eyes with pleasant thoughts of the silent forest and wonderful new friends. Also, I was thankful Lynn had talked me into coming to Alaska for a fresh start after my serious problems in Seattle.

I fell asleep wondering why my ER Board registration hadn't arrived. I hoped there was no issue related to my bogus probation status the last month before I completed ER training.

Chapter 10 Flying

The warmer weather and longer days of spring provided great flying opportunities. The brighter days brought more energy to recharge my batteries dulled by the long winter nights. Some patients spoke to me about wintertime depression, but that was not a problem for me. I liked my job, enjoyed my new friends, and even joined Ed mushing dogs on the trails behind his home. I found a fixed-base operator on Merrill Field that offered aircraft rental and flight lessons. I called Ed and Lucille one morning to tell them I planned to do some flying and thought it would be fun to fly out to Wasilla for a visit.

"Circle over the house. We'll listen for you and meet you at the airstrip."

Over coffee and a sticky bun, Ed said, "I'll go flying with you any time. Let's plan a day when the weather is good to the east, and I'll show you my bear-hunting shack out at St. Anne Lake."

"Count me out, Kelly," Lucille said. "I don't know how I've lasted this long in Alaska. I won't go out in a canoe, let alone get in an airplane. Good thing I enjoy cooking for everyone. That's where I get my fun."

After a flight to Talkeetna about 90 miles north, I returned to Merrill, where I found Dale Ayers visiting in the flight office. "Hey, sweet Kelly. How are you? Are you getting back into flying more?"

His friendly greeting infuriated me. I had not forgiven him for his indiscretions in McGrath. "Now that winter is leaving, I took your suggestion to get back in the air."

"I called yesterday to tell you about a Maule for sale here at Merrill. I heard the owner had a heart attack and isn't flying anymore." He got up and looked out the window. "I'll drive you over to it. I thought you might want to look at it, but Lynn said you were sleeping. Do you have time now?"

"Sure."

Dale headed for the door. "They have a leaseback Super Cub here at the flight school. You could take a few lessons and get your taildragger endorsement. It's a perfect trainer."

I turned in my rental keys.

Dale opened the door and held it for me. "Let's go kick some tires."

We walked to his filthy Ford Bronco and got in. He drove the perimeter road of the airport in deep ruts of icy mud and then onto black asphalt, steamy from the spring sun.

I commented, "Look at the rows and rows of taildraggers. In Arlington, north of Seattle, they used Maules to tow gliders. I don't think I saw a Super Cub the whole time I was in Washington State."

"No use for Super Cubs down there. They're slow. Cruise is only a hundred, and with paved runways everywhere, you don't need one. They're made for Alaska's dirt strips and bush flying."

"Here it is." Dale stopped in front of a yellow Maule. "Let's get out and look at it. I talked to the guy. He's sad about losing his medical certification."

We looked at it as carefully as we could without removing the wing covers. "It looks great to me. I'd like to talk to the guy."

"I checked prices. He's ready to sell. You won't get a better plane for the price. Not much time on the engine."

"Still, it sounds like a lot to me, but I make good money and could swing it with a short-term loan."

"The guy told me he'd be in Seattle for a couple weeks visiting his daughter. I asked him to call me when he gets back. When he returns, we can take the covers off and look inside. I don't like to touch the plane without him being here."

Dale dropped me back at my car. "Thanks for telling me about the plane. Let me know when he gets back. I'll schedule time with an instructor in the Super Cub, so I can get checked out and endorsed. Thanks." I started to slam the heavy door on his four-by-four. He held up his hand to stop me.

"No, Kelly, thank you for not telling Lynn. I appreciate it. I got checked out medically, and I'm clean. I'd never forgive myself if I gave her something."

"You're welcome." I closed the door and watched him drive away, still disgusted by his behavior.

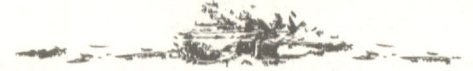

Work, taking taildragger lessons, and studying for the Boards sped the month of March into April. *Breakup,* the Alaskan term for the coming of spring, arrived. Melting snow turned streets into creeks and back yards into swamps. Ice-covered lakes and streams cracked. Large chunks washed ashore and finally melted. The ground cover of white turned to dirty white and then gray. Piles of junk in yards around town, gracefully buried and out of view for months, become eyesores once again. According to newspaper reports, occasionally the disappearing snow even uncovered a body.

The melt lasted for a couple of weeks. Standing water slowly seeped into the soggy ground. One of the nurses went hiking and found wildflowers popping up at the edge of mountain snow.

Lynn and I looked forward to our trip to Seattle, even if it was for a grueling exam. With both of us being gone from the ER at the same time for a week, the other docs whined. I reassured Andy Enders, one of the ER docs, an avid fisherman and hunter who always seemed to be taking time off, "Remember, we're not going for fun like you usually do. This is serious business."

"Yeah, tell me about it. We're slaving. Up to our elbows in Alaskan alligators, and you're picking daffodils in Seattle."

I placed many phone calls to check the status of my test application and to find out why it hadn't been confirmed. I still hadn't received anything in writing when we went to the airport. I told Lynn my concerns. "Don't worry about it. Yours was probably delivered to Alabama—they get AK and AL mixed up sometimes. It'll be there in Seattle and confirmed when we register. They cashed your check, didn't they?"

"I don't remember seeing it."

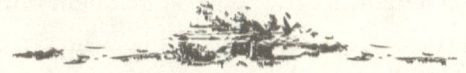

Our flight was okay leaving Anchorage and along the coastline. However, when we were at the Canada-United States border, we suddenly hit clear air turbulence. There were still a few trays and glasses out. The plane dropped, bottomed out hard, and the pilot's voice came on the intercom. "This is unexpected turbulence. Flight attendants, passengers, take your seats and fasten your seat belts." Before he finished speaking, more hard rocking threw me into Lynn, who bumped the side of the plane near her window.

Trays hit the floor. Overhead compartments flew open. Small bags and other projectiles rained down on passengers. Looking down the aisle ahead of us, people ducked and hung on to ride out the bumping and rocking movements.

Lynn looked pale. "Just hang on. I've been through worse than this. Flying into Boston during a nor'easter was hell. Much worse than this, with blinding rain."

A flight attendant near me gripped her seat and looked worried. Spilled milk in the aisle first rolled toward me, then away, back and forth, as the plane was thrown around by unseen forces. The smell of vomit from a nearby seat stunk up the air.

After what seemed like a very long time, the pilot's calm voice came on the intercom. "Sorry we had such a rough ride. Air Traffic Control said it should be smooth ahead at this altitude, so you can all relax. Flight attendants are free to move about the cabin. Passengers are requested to remain seated and belted until I turn the seat belt light off."

A loud voice called out, "Relax, shit. Who can relax after a ride like that? Just somebody bring me a drink."

Laughter broke out at his comment, which lightened the atmosphere.

A light rain welcomed us to Seattle. We picked up our rental car and headed to the Sheraton to check in. Staying at the location of the test, with two days to rest and socialize, would provide us the least hassle possible for the important exam.

Chapter 11 Boards

The morning of the exam, Lynn and I showered before the wake-up call and headed downstairs to the claustrophobic hotel coffee shop for breakfast. The room was packed with people crowded in booths and around small tables.

We found two larger tables with a few chairs unoccupied. Someone waved and motioned us to join them. There were a few we knew well from our class of eight. Claustrophobic feelings arose in me. Fear struck without warning. I turned blindly to escape and bumped square into Lynn.

She grabbed my arms. "Kelly, what is it?"

"Being here. I have to get outside."

"Get ahold of yourself. It's a panic attack. It'll pass. Now stop it." She pinched my arm and twisted.

The pain stopped my accelerating panic.

I buried my fear. My pounding heart slowed. We sat at a table with a friend. "Kelly, you're looking good. Maybe a little too skinny. How are you doing?"

"Good in Alaska. Anchorage hasn't been as serene as I thought it would, but being back in Seattle for the first time since all my problems the last year of residency has set me on edge."

"You're not the only one. I think it's the anticipation of finally taking the exam."

I picked up a menu. Nothing looked good. "I hate tests. My anxiety level goes way up." The waitress took my pancake order.

Lynn studied my face. "Smile, Kelly. You, of all people, have nothing to fear with tests."

I faked a smile.

One of the others at the table asked, "So, Lynn, are you glad you went to Alaska?"

"It's the best thing I've ever done. You all will have to come up for a visit."

One of the guys announced, "Suppose you heard, Kelly's old flame, Brett Warren, got back on drugs again. Good thing you got out of that relationship when you did, Kelly. He was in rehab for the second time and walked out."

I looked at him blankly, trying to process the information quickly.

Lynn covered for me. "We've had no contact with him. He's the last person on earth Kelly wants to see. He's caused her enough pain."

"Sorry I mentioned it, but I heard he went to Alaska. I thought you should know that, Kelly. I don't know what his mental state is."

After my order arrived, I watched my thick pancakes, soft and gooey in the middle, slowly absorb the cold syrup like large, round, inedible sponges. I sipped coffee and tried to listen to the conversation, but my thoughts distracted me. I wanted to be home in Minnesota, sitting at the table with my mother and sister, eating my mother's light, thin, delicious hotcakes with hot maple syrup, syrup made painstakingly by Aunt Irene, and talking about fishing and the weather, non-threatening things. Brett's name wouldn't surface.

Chairs backed away from the table. People left. I looked at my watch. It was past the time for registration. Lynn handed me my coffee. "Drink the last of this and wake up. If you aren't going to eat those pancakes, eat my English muffin. You need something in your stomach before you start the exam."

I followed her suggestion, and we took our places outside the testing conference room, following the signs. Alphabetical markers pointed to the proper line to join based on the first letter of our last names. I joined the M-N-O-Ps, the last one in line and at the table, placing my ID and driver's license in front of a raven-like woman with a prominent nose and shiny dyed black hair drawn so tightly into a bun that it gave her a face lift. Reading glasses sat on her pointed nose, secured around her neck with a decorative silver and black beaded chain. She studied my picture ID and then her list. She looked up at me and nervously removed her glasses as if to see me better.

"Dr. McKay?"

"Yes."

"I don't have you on my final list. Did you think you were to take the Emergency Medicine Board Exam?"

"Yes. I completed the residency at Harbor Medical Center here in Seattle and sent everything in along with the fee at the same time my roommate Lynn Cabot did. She got her verification before we left Alaska, but I did not." I tried to remain calm. My hands were cold and sweaty. "I called and left many messages but hadn't received a call back from the exam office before we left."

What if I can't take it after all this?

"Well, Doctor, you're not on the list. I can't let you enter the examination room."

"There's a mistake. Can't you check with someone?"

She raised her eyebrows. Her narrow-set eyes, exaggerated with heavy black eye liner, peered back at me, angry, as if I was asking her to do something unreasonable. Her artificially penciled eyebrows arched sharply. "This is very irregular. If you are not on the list, you can't take the test."

When she stood, I saw her thin upper body was bound to earth by the gravitational pull on a voluminous butt that nearly toppled her chair. She caught the chair with her left hand. "Dr. McKay. You wait right there." Her tone suggested she was afraid I would commandeer a chair in the exam room. I'll see Mr. Carlston. He's in charge."

Her hips tilted with each rapid step toward a tall man who looked like an overseer.

He shook his head and followed her as she walked back toward me.

I watched everyone else in line enter small privacy cubicles for proper vetting. There, digital photos were taken to confirm identity before the tech made an image of an infrared venous scan of one palm for additional security for entry on each of the six testing days. Only those properly vetted would be allowed to take the grueling tests that ended with an oral exam.

The large double doors clicked shut, leaving only me waiting.

"Hello, Dr. McKay. Elsie tells me you *thought* you were taking the Emergency Medicine Boards today."

"I sent in the application and money. She says I'm not on the list."

"I remember your application very well, Dr. McKay. You should know that we verify all the details on such an important application. There are certain criteria that are mandatory. Your residency program data listed you as not completing the program and being placed on probation your last year. We couldn't possibly allow you to take the Boards. Did you think you could slip that past us? The first requirement is that you must have completed a residency, and you, apparently, did not."

"That information is wrong. Why wasn't I notified of this?"

"I'm sure we did."

"I want to take the exam today. It's my right to do it. I have completed the requirements. I sent the registration fee in many months ago. Did anyone call the program and check?"

"It's done by a committee of people. I imagine someone called."

"Dr. Jackson Hunter is the residency director. I completed the program here in Seattle at Harbor Medical Center. If I call him and he verifies that everything is in order, then will you let me take the exam?"

"This has never happened before. I will not take anyone's verbal okay. If you are to be qualified, I must have everything in writing. The exam is beginning now. I think you'll have to be satisfied with taking it another time. It will be offered again next year."

"I flew in from Alaska to take it. It's your screw-up. I'll call the program director right now. Will I find you here at the registration desk?"

"Yes," was his simple reply. He stood tall and straight as if he were exercising military authority, spun on his heel, and walked away.

Elsie smiled approvingly at his back.

I punched in the main hospital number on my cell. The familiar husky voice of a telephone operator who'd been there a hundred years answered. "Harbor Medical Center. How may I direct your call?"

"Hi, Hazel, it's Kelly McKay. I need to talk to Dr. Hunter. Can you find him for me?"

"Oh, Kelly. How are you? We miss you."

"I'm fine now. I'm in town to take the Boards, and they're telling me the records show I didn't finish the residency."

"That's terrible after all you went through. I'll find him. He'll make it right."

Mindless music filled the void as I waited for him to answer his page. I just hoped he was in.

Finally, he answered, "Hunter here."

"Dr. Hunter, it's Kelly McKay."

"Kelly, how nice of you to call. I was hoping I'd get to see you. I knew you'd be in town for the Boards."

"That's why I'm calling you. I'm at the Sheraton. They're blocking me from the exam. Their records show I was on probation and didn't finish the residency."

"Dammit! I asked administration to sanitize your probation file and inform the National Data Bank that all negative information about losing hospital staff privileges should be expunged. I'm so sorry, Kelly. What can we do at this point?"

"The guy in charge here said he wouldn't let me take the exam without having written documents from you. Can I get them now? I want to get in there and take the test today, otherwise I have to wait months."

"Sure, I'll do it immediately."

"Lynn and I have a rental car. I could probably be at the hospital in fifteen minutes."

"You sit tight. I'll get your file and drive there myself and talk to them. I'm really sorry. Heads will roll over this. Those incompetents! I told them how important it was to clear you completely."

I walked back to the registration area. The door guard refused me entry. Carlston was nowhere to be seen. I asked the guard, "Did the tall man here a few minutes ago, Mr. Carlston, say where he was going?"

"I think he took all those ladies working at the tables for coffee. There's a break in the testing after one hour. I'm sure they'll be back here by then."

I went back to the couch along the wall near registration and hunkered down to wait.

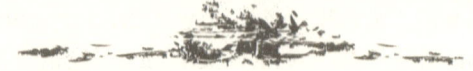

Someone touched my arm. I opened my eyes and couldn't immediately make out the features of the back-lighted male figure in front of me. He held out a hand. It was Hunter. "You took a little nap. Glad I found you. I forgot to ask exactly where you were."

"Oh, Dr. Hunter. Thanks for coming.

"I've known Carlston for years. He acts like an inflexible jerk. I already talked to him and gave him the required documents. He's scrutinizing them now. I think he'll let you in."

Hunter pulled me to my feet. "You look good. How are you feeling?"

"Fine, until I got here."

"After all you've been through, this is just a speed bump." He hesitated and then, in his usual blunt manner, said, "Warren's on the loose again. Have you seen him?"

"Not since I was in ICU on a vent."

"I have no firsthand information but was told he bailed out of rehab and was going to Alaska. I just heard yesterday and would have called you but thought I might see you here, just not quite like this."

Carlston interrupted. "Dr. McKay. Your papers are in order. You may take the exam beginning with the second hour. I will remain late at the end of the day and monitor you during the first section you missed."

Hunter responded, "Great, Charles. Thanks for being so flexible." Winking at me, he said, "Kelly is a great doctor. I have to get back to the hospital and do a talk for the medical students on street drugs at noon." He turned to me. "I wish you were here to do it for me. I like the guy that got your chief resident job, but he doesn't have your talent."

"Thanks for coming in my time of need. Lynn and I will stop by the hospital to visit when we are done with the exam on Saturday. We want to see everyone."

Hunter rushed off, and Carlston started me on the detailed process of verifying my identification and eligibility to sit for the exam. Lynn and I had reviewed the process, but the added stress of not being allowed to register rattled my confidence and spiked my anxiety. After I showed my photo ID, they took a digital photo and did my infrared vein scan. After all the hassle, I was shocked Carlston let me take the exam, starting right after the first break.

When the double doors swung open for the exodus of the test takers, I spotted Lynn searching the crowd, presumably for me. I waved.

She pushed her way through the throng to me. "Kelly, where were you? I didn't see you in there."

I told her of my crisis and the resolution.

Lynn just shook her head. "I thought you had a panic attack and bolted. At least you got it all straightened out. Tonight, I'll buy you an extra dry Sapphire martini. You'll need it by then. The first section of the exam was brutal."

The test takers were from across the United States. We knew a few of them from our program and from meeting them at conferences. Throughout the week of the Boards, six days of testing for six hours per day, we were barely functional. Instead of going to Harbor ER for a visit, each night we ate well, went to bed early, and discussed a few fine points in some of the questions. We knew the tests varied and that it was unlikely we'd both had the same series of questions. After the oral interrogation, we compared notes and decided Dr. Hunter had prepared us well for the exam by burning us during the morning pyres.

At the end of the last day, Saturday, we sat in the hotel bar and celebrated with other exhausted ER docs. Hunter had come through at the last minute to save me from missing the exam, but he'd lost my respect when he had abandoned me the previous year. With Brett Warren on the loose, I felt safest in the bar with my back against the wall. I'd learned that from my friend Cy Jones, a Seattle Police Department detective.

The next morning, Lynn and I drove to Harbor. It would have been nice to arrive at 7 a.m. for the morning pyre and see more people at change of shift. Instead, we arrived about nine, drank bad coffee, and hung out at the nursing desk for a while.

Hunter wasn't there. The nurses introduced us to Dr. Alexander, the chief resident who was now sharing responsibilities with Hunter. I recognized him from the day of the interviews, the one whose wife got a dermatology position. I asked him about Dr. Hunter. He said, "I run things pretty much the same as before, but he actually takes some time off, mostly evenings." Alexander pulled back his white coat, revealing an array of devices hooked to his belt.

"Hunter gives me all his beepers—for the fixed-wing flight and helicopter services and Medic 1. He still carries a cell phone, but we try not to bother him."

I smiled. "That's hard to believe he isn't sleeping with his radios anymore. He's probably in withdrawal without being on call 24/7."

A couple of residents made positive comments. One of them took me aside to say Hunter had actually gone into a slump and had been less communicative with staff after I left town. The department had calmed down, though, and they felt Alexander was doing a good job as chief resident.

Lynn said, "Maybe Hunter is feeling a little remorse for not defending Kelly."

Dr. Alexander walked over to our group and heard Lynn's remark. "You're right. I'm glad you got to see him, Kelly. He was horrified you had to experience yet another issue when they wouldn't let you into the exam. He was furious."

"Well, it's over now. It feels good to be able to leave town."

Lynn added, "Yes, but we have to wait three months to get the results."

Just after noon, we walked back to our rental car and headed to the hotel for our luggage en route to catching our flight home.

Chapter 12 Back to Alaska

Early flowers filled the hotel's gardens. Mount Rainier came out from beneath a spring mist to bid us farewell and remind us that one nice day in Seattle made up for thirty rainy ones. We barely made it to the airport in time to board our flight home.

The Alaska Airlines jet took off from Sea-Tac toward the south, and, before falling asleep, we got a close view of glistening snowfields on the west side of the silent volcano.

Back in Alaska, the giant snow scape was awakening from its long winter. The touchdown in Anchorage was smooth.

We exited with the throng of fliers who looked like people heading home after a vacation away from winter weather. Returning Alaskans have that special look: sunburned, wearing leis, jeans, and hiking boots, and carrying frame backpacks with ratty parkas and sleeping bags tied on them. Half the passengers looked Alaskan. The other half looked like lawyers returning from business trips Outside.

Dale stood in the baggage area leaning against a wall. Lynn gave him a bear-hug. "Have you been waiting long?"

He reeked of alcohol.

"Your flight's late. I came out early and ran into a buddy from my helicopter logging camp days in southeast Alaska. We had a few drinks. His flight left just before yours landed. The timing was perfect. You girls want a drink?"

I shook my head, "I think I'd rather head home. I have to work tonight, so I need to unpack and rest. If you two want to have food or a drink, just drop me off at the apartment."

Dale looked at Lynn.

"Food sounds good to me. Are you sure you don't want to join us, Kelly?"

"Yeah. I think I'll nap. After the Boards and the partying, I'm really tired."

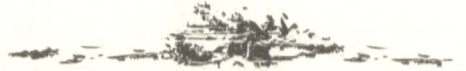

I placed my luggage next to a basket of dirty clothes and scanned the refrigerator. After the tasteless airline snack, yogurt and a stale rice cake satisfied my appetite enough to let me sleep. When I got up, I found a note from Lynn on the dining room table near the sliding door to the deck. *There's take-out Chinese food in the refrigerator for you to zap for dinner. I'll see you in the morning. I work at seven. Lynn.*

This was a pleasant surprise. After eating, I set off for the hospital early. A whoosh of the ambulance door announced my entrance. Nurses gathered around the desk talking to Dewey Churchill, an ER doctor who looked eager to leave. His jacket and a small backpack sat on the desk ready for his escape.

"Hi, Dewey. You aren't anxious to leave, are you?"

He picked up his pack and headed toward me. "Am I glad to see you. Thanks for getting here early. I cleared out the ER for you." He slung the pack over a shoulder. "I'm flying out to Iliamna. The salmon are running, and the bears are already fishing. I work as a doctor only to support my photography habit. Those bears are awesome."

"When are you leaving?"

"Daybreak, if the weather holds."

"Be careful."

He smiled and was gone.

One of the nurses said, "Dewey met a lady pilot with a float plane. He hasn't been able to stop talking about this trip all night. How was Seattle?"

"I'm glad to be back. The Boards were hard, but it was good to see friends."

The new shift of nurses arrived, among them Vic and Rob. Our uneventful night changed about 3 a.m. when a teenage male with abdominal pain arrived with his parents. Vic checked him in. "Kelly, this one looks like appendicitis to me. Want to make a bet?"

"Do I get to examine him first?"

"Oh, all right."

I looked at the ER record. Timothy T. Lawson III. Why does that name sound familiar?

Tim, age 16, appeared flushed and sweaty. A woman, presumably his mother, wiped his forehead with a tissue. A tall, good-looking blond male, an older image of Tim, stood at the side of Tim's bed gripping the side rail. Young Tim looked up when I walked up to his bed. "Hi, Tim, I'm Dr. McKay. Vic, your nurse, tells me you are having abdominal pain."

He started to speak, but his father interrupted. "I want a surgeon called, now. My son has appendicitis."

I stiffened, taking an immediate dislike to the man. A power figure. In control. Doesn't want to deal with any woman. Won't let his son speak.

"Did you call a surgeon before you came in, sir?"

"No, but I want one called now."

"I'm responsible for all patients who present to the ER until another physician assumes care. Our procedure is to evaluate all patients and then call in a specialist as needed. A surgeon would certainly want blood work done, so your son's care can be started right away."

"Get on with it then."

I turned back to Tim. His mother gripped the boy's hand. "When did you start feeling ill, Tim?"

"Two days ago while playing basketball, I had a little pain in my right side. I thought I pulled a muscle. I took some ibuprofen, and it went away. Since yesterday, every step I take jars my side. The pain got worse after I ate breakfast. I came home from school early and went to bed. When I woke up, it was real bad."

I asked him a few more questions and examined him. "I agree with your dad, Tim. You have a fever, almost 101, and your exam suggests appendicitis. We'll need to check your urine and do a blood test. We'll start an IV and give you something for pain."

"Thank you, Doctor," Tim said in a quiet voice. He looked to his mother for reassurance.

His dad stepped up to the bed. "Buck up, Tim. Unless they're incompetent, it'll only take them one stick for the blood and IV. I'll be here watching after you."

When I arrived at the desk, Vic was waiting for me. "I should have warned you, Kelly. That is Timothy T. Lawson the third, son of Timothy T. Lawson the second, grandson of Timothy Lawson the first. The father and grandfather are famous malpractice lawyers in Anchorage. Isn't the father a pleasant man?"

"I'll pay you back, Vic."

He laughed. "Well, what do you think, Doc?"

"I'm with you. He has appendicitis. I guess the bet is off." I wrote some orders. "Once you get the IV in, you can give him a couple milligrams of morphine. Who's on for surgery?"

Vic looked at the call schedule. "This is going to be a bad scene. It's Dr. Wells."

Rob said, "Oh, shit. I hope I get a flight and don't have to be around for this."

"Okay, what's the problem with Wells?"

Vic sat down by me. "The Lawsons have sued many of the doctors in Anchorage over the past twenty years, and he comes in here thinking a doctor will jump to his commands because of his power. Well, his wife is a divorce lawyer. It couldn't be any worse. Tim Lawson the second sued Wells for malpractice about a year ago. Mrs. Lawson represented Wells' wife in his divorce. Wells was the doctor that the video caught in the garage with the nurse."

"Well, I'm new around here. I'll play dumb. I'll call Wells and just tell him I've got a hot one and let him deal with it."

"Good luck. Wells is a dynamic, volatile surgeon. He's good and knows it." Rob added more to Vic's story. "He is also good looking and uses his looks to his advantage. He lost big with both the malpractice case and in the divorce. His nurse says he's become bitter and talks about quitting surgery because of liability risks."

Wells arrived about twenty minutes after my call. I handed him Tim's blood work. "His white count just came back at eighteen thousand."

He picked up the chart and disappeared into the patient room.

Vic switched on the video-audio monitor in Tim's room. The aggressive exchange between the two professionals was embarrassing to watch. Wells' final statement was, "No, I will not operate on your son." He stormed out of the room.

Lawson followed on his heels, yelling, "I'll sue you for patient abandonment! You cannot refuse to take care of this boy—he could die."

Wells responded, "You should have thought of that when you sued every fucking doctor in the state. Go to Seattle for your care. They won't know you there."

Wells threw the chart on the desk. "As the new doctor in town, I'm sorry you are caught in the middle of this. Both of Tim's parents have sued me. I cannot, in good conscience, be his surgeon. You'll have a helluva time finding anyone who will."

Tim Lawson II wedged his imposing figure between Wells and me. "You can't refuse to take care of him. Under federal law, you'll be charged with a COBRA violation, and I'll see that it's worse than that. It comes out of your personal funds, not malpractice. It will hurt worse if you pay it yourself."

"Oh, I'm not that dumb, Lawson. I'll document this very well. Your son will receive treatment, stabilization, and antibiotics, and he will be taken care of by a surgeon . . . but not by me. I know that law better than you do. Now, if you'll excuse me, we have work to do."

Lawson stormed away from the desk and back to Tim's room. I heard Mrs. Lawson's distressed voice. "I knew this would happen. We should have just hopped on a flight like we've done before."

Wells' external jugulars were so distended they were pulsing. His face was red and his hand trembled as he dialed the phone. "I was having a nice evening till this. You'll have to find another surgeon."

"I'm really sorry. That is a terrible problem." I dialed many numbers and talked to four general surgeons in Anchorage. When they learned who the patient was and that Wells wouldn't take the case, all of them turned me down.

"I struck out, Dr. Wells. No one will touch him."

Wells sat at the desk, head down. "Get antibiotics running on the kid right away and make him comfortable. Check to see if fixed wing is available to fly him to Fairbanks. I'll start calling up there."

Rob dialed the pilot. I looked up the Fairbanks hospital number and dialed while Wells dictated a note and wrote in the chart. I asked who was on call for surgery in Fairbanks and got his number. I paged him to our ER. When he called, I handed the phone to Wells.

While Wells was talking, I called our on-call administrator. "I have a bad situation here. I wanted to inform you because it could come back to haunt all of us, especially if anything goes wrong with the patient. He is really a nice kid. Clinically, he has appendicitis. Our interventions here would qualify as stabilization. The care is available here, but we just can't get a surgeon to operate on him. Wells is on the phone with a surgeon in Fairbanks, and I think we will be flying him there for care."

"I'll come down. It'll take me about fifteen minutes to get to the hospital. Thanks for letting me know."

When the administrator walked in, Wells exclaimed, "Look what the cat dragged in. Lawson call you too?"

"No, Kelly did. This puts the hospital in a terrible situation. This may be a COBRA violation. I think you should reconsider. I think you should operate on him."

"I can't. The new guy in Fairbanks just accepted him. We're shipping him north."

I hated being involved in this bad scenario. "What if Tim deteriorates en route? He could become septic and die."

"Dr. McKay, that's a terrible thought. I can see the headlines, now. 'Local doctor refuses care, lawyers' son dies.' Why don't you ride along with him? That way he'll have a doctor by his side. He isn't being abandoned—shit—we even sent a doctor along for the ride. That'll stand up in court."

Rob hung up the phone. "Fixed wing is available. They're looking for a pilot. The one on duty is off on a personal trip in the morning. He's getting a replacement to cover for this flight since it would put him into overtime and possibly make him miss his vacation flight."

The administrator looked worried, pacing. "Are you willing to fly with him to Fairbanks, Kelly? I'll get another ER doc to come in and cover the rest of your shift."

"I don't mind. I'll call Lynn. She'll come in a couple hours early. She's on in the morning anyway. It's 4:30 now. It'll just take her a few minutes to get here."

The administrator sounded relieved. "Okay. Wells, why don't you and McKay go in and explain the plan? I'll try to stay out of it."

Wells took a deep breath and stood. Rob joined us. The Lawsons were not happy but knew there was no obvious loophole. They wanted to ride on the flight with us. Rob explained, "We're weight limited. We can take one of you. There are frequent commercial flights if you want to check with the airlines."

Mr. Lawson snarled, "I'll go with Tim to make sure everything is done right." He looked at me. "I want him in no pain." He emphasized, louder, "No pain."

Tim's searching eyes avoided his father's stare and tracked from his mother's eyes to mine. "Doctor, I get air sick. Would you give me some medicine so I don't throw up? I hate to throw up."

His mother cut in, "Of course she will, Tim." She squeezed his hand. "You're going to do just fine, Son. We can visit my sister when you get out of the hospital. Stay with her a couple days till you feel like traveling. They might want you to stay in Fairbanks about a week to get your stitches out."

Tim's groggy eyes brightened. "I like Aunt Gini. Would you call and tell her we're flying up? Maybe she'll come to the hospital. Dad, you're so busy, you don't have time to come along. Why don't you just let Mom come. I'll be fine."

"If that's the way you feel, Tim, okay. I have a very important conference this morning. Mother can go and call me. I always carry my cell phone. Are you sure, Tim?"

Tim was obviously relieved. "Yes, Dad."

During our ambulance ride to International, Rob, Tim, and I rode in the back and Mrs. Lawson sat in front with the driver. Mr. Lawson tailgated us. He parked quickly and stood at the perimeter fence until we taxied to the active runway.

We gave Tim IV medication for pain and nausea. Rob monitored him throughout the flight. Tim and his mother both slept. Before closing her eyes, she apologized for her husband. "He is so compulsive and competitive. He doesn't have much time for us. His clients always come first." Her loving eyes looked at Tim. "He cares a lot for his son, but I was surprised he offered to go with him. I think he forgot about his work commitments this morning."

I nodded but said nothing.

She continued, "I'll call my office at nine and tell them I won't be in for a few days. I can handle some pressing things by phone." She looked at her resting son and whispered. "Do you think he'll do all right?"

"He should do fine. Recently, appendectomies are being done by laparoscopy. Not much cutting and the recovery is rapid."

The flight was smooth, but the hard landing at Fairbanks awakened Tim with a jolt. His bleary eyes scanned the inside of the plane, and his initial confusion changed to awareness. "That was good medicine, I didn't puke."

A waiting ambulance carried us to Dr. Stein at the hospital's ER. The young dark-haired man with a quick smile hit it off with Tim immediately. Mrs. Lawson stood back and didn't interfere. Her sister, a plump woman with similar features but older and fatter, arrived in a flurry and laid effusive kisses on Tim. I was relieved to leave Tim and his mother in good hands.

Rob and I were on our way out to the ambulance for a ride back to the airport when Mrs. Lawson caught up to us. "Tim wanted me to tell you thanks. I thank you, too, for being considerate under such difficult circumstances."

On the way back to the airport, Rob looked distressed. "Kelly, did you see our pilot?"

"I got a glimpse of the back of their heads. Looked like Dale and that new guy."

"It was Dale Ayers and Ted, the ex-military guy with the crewcut. He's fixed wing only, not helicopter rated. Dale's licensed in everything it seems, at least that's what he says, but he doesn't fly fixed wing very often."

I thought back on the hard landing. "I wonder who was doing the flying. This King Air almost bounced. It woke Tim up from a drugged sleep."

"I know. That's what I was getting to. I hope I'm wrong, but when I went up front to ask Dale something, he reeked of alcohol. I think I've smelled it on him before. I think he chews gum and wears powerful aftershave to cover it up. Do you know if he has a drinking problem, Kelly? He worries me."

Rob's words shot a jolt of fear into me. Shit. Am I gonna lie and cover up for him? "I don't know, Rob. I don't think so. Lynn has never complained to me about it."

We climbed into the back of the big aircraft. It rumbled alive and soon was airborne. How does it feel, Kelly, flying with a drunk? You know he has a problem. You've seen it before. Are you going to do something about it before he kills someone?

Chapter 13 Dale's Drinking

We didn't get back to Anchorage that morning until nine. Dale gave Rob and me a ride back from the airport. They dropped me off at the apartment. I wanted to go directly home to bed. I was exhausted because the first night shift after being off is always more difficult for me. My biological clock was set to staying awake during the day. Even the long nap before I went to work didn't help much. I set my alarm for 6 p.m.

Dale and Rob went on to the hospital, where Rob had his car. Dale was on flight call until 5 p.m. Regulations required pilots cover no more than twelve hours. If the pilot's shift ended at a port away from home, they had to take a twelve-hour break. That can be an inconvenience for everyone at times.

Dale said he was going back to the hospital helicopter call room in the hangar adjacent to the hospital to sleep.

After a restless sleep with frequent awakenings and thoughts of Tim and of Dale's drinking, I was back at the hospital.

I felt like I had never left.

The waiting room was full, the rooms were full, and the nurses were cranky. Lynn had four admissions that she had to finish. It took her two additional hours. When she finished, I followed her outside to tell her my concerns about Dale.

She blew up and yelled in my face. I had never seen her behave like this before. Luckily, the automated doors closed behind us. Her wrath wasn't heard indoors, but if anyone was watching the surveillance camera, I'm sure her angry mannerisms and facial expressions were obvious.

"Lynn, I was close to Dale on the flight to Fairbanks. He smelled of booze. When did he quit drinking yesterday? Did he spend the night with you? Do you know when his last drink was?"

She stomped her foot. "Kelly, don't be falsely accusing Dale of drinking on the job. He would never do that, and you know it. He loves his job. You tried to lay it on me about him drinking and flying before. It just wouldn't happen! He left me about midnight and didn't drink after dinner."

"Well, Lynn, he smelled strong, not just a whiff, not like it was left over from hours ago. I hate to tell you this, but Rob asked me about it. He said he's smelled it before. If you don't do something now, I will have to go to administration. If he doesn't hurt someone with his drunk driving, he's gonna crash an aircraft." I begged her, "Lynn, you have to talk to him."

She stormed off.

When Lynn returned at 6:30 a.m. to take over again, I was happy to see her because it meant I could go home. I was concerned about how she'd react after our confrontation.

Lynn walked in, went directly to the locker room, donned a scrub suit, and presented herself. "Well, give me some work. I'm ready to roll."

I told her lightly, "Be glad you were home sleeping. It got very weird overnight with three overdoses, then two borderline personalities cutting themselves. One of them had at least a hundred healed wounds from previous slashes on both arms. The patient explained to me that she had so much emotional pain, the only way to relieve it was with physical pain. She said, 'I feel better with the sharp pain. Seeing the blood helps. Then, I get scared and don't want to die so I call 9-1-1.'"

Lynn growled, "I have no patience for psych stuff."

"We also saw a teenager with a racing heart, hyperventilating. She was frightened after taking six packages of Mini Thin stimulants. Duh. I really wanted to go home at that point. I'm happy you're here, in case you haven't noticed."

"See you in the morning, Kelly. Dale's at the apartment watching the morning news. I thought you might want to join him for breakfast. I told him I'd eat at the hospital."

I frowned. She gave me a look I have never seen on her before, kind of a funny half-smile that said wait and see. I wasn't sure what it meant. I walked home slowly, trying to decide what I should say to him.

My brisk walk in the moist morning air reminded me of fall in Seattle. A clinging dampness made the sun feel cold, but it turned drops of moisture on shrubs to pinpoint diamonds. It was broad daylight, yet on my way home, I developed the uneasy feeling that someone was following me.

In Seattle, I always carried pepper spray in my hand, concealed in a pocket. I had never felt threatened walking through Anchorage or alone along the route to the hospital, except by moose.

I tried to look around inconspicuously. I checked behind me. About a block back, a couple walked hand in hand. I had seen no one near the hospital when I left. I thought I was anxious because of the crazies in the ER and having to confront Dale now. Why me?

I made a noisy entrance when I dropped the little backpack I carry as a purse. It hit the metal screen door. When I opened the door, Dale was sipping coffee. He looked spiffed up. Not quite what I expected. Not an empty beer can in sight.

"Hi, Kelly. I haven't had much time to talk to you since you got back from Seattle. I have great news. I got ahold of the old guy with the Maule. He's back in town. I went out and looked the plane over in detail, including the logbooks. Not many hours on the engine because he hasn't been able to fly much since the engine had a complete overhaul. If you're still interested, we better tell him. There's another guy looking at it today."

"Thanks for taking your time to do all that, Dale. I'm definitely interested."

"Why don't you sleep on it and I'll pick you up and take you out to look at it again? If you think you want it, I'll have a mechanic go over it. It will cost a hundred smackers, but it's worth it to get a professional opinion. He's a guy I'd trust with my life."

"I do need to sleep after the stupid night I just put in. Where will you be about three?"

"I'm on backup call. You can reach me on the beeper and the cell phone. I could be on a flight. Otherwise, I'll pick you up when you call and we'll go out to Merrill."

He sounded excited. When he talked fast, he lost most of his Southern accent. At 8 a.m., I doubted he'd been drinking. Sometimes he was a likeable guy. I understood Lynn's defending him. Maybe it was my imagination that he'd been drinking and flying. He was garrulous, Southern, and crude. Maybe the combination wasn't a good mix.

He asked if I wanted to go out for breakfast. I declined. Sleep sounded better. I invited him to stay for granola and yogurt. For some reason, he said he'd rather eat dirt and laughed loudly on his way out.

I pulled the drapes and checked the deck door and the front door to be sure they were locked.

In the bedroom, just as I was getting ready to put in my foam earplugs and turn on the fan, I thought I heard footsteps outside the back door. I got up quietly and listened. I heard a car pass, and then the helicopter took off from the hospital helipad and flew overhead, shaking the building. I closed the bedroom door, making it nearly pitch dark in the room. I locked the bedroom door.

I never did that. Why am I doing this?

It had been a weird night.

I tried to avoid the real thought that was bothering me. In Seattle, they told us Brett Warren had gone to Alaska. I wondered if he was in Anchorage. Would he follow me here? Was he watching me?

Chapter 14 Buying a Plane

Dale picked me up that afternoon and we drove the short distance to Merrill Field. After removing the wing covers, we carefully examined the surfaces. "The paint looks great to me, but the doors are strange."

"It's a useful variation. They're gull-wing doors that flip up. The owner had a business flying photographers." Dale unlocked the door on the pilot's side and then leaned across and popped open the one on the passenger side. "They can be left open in flight to get some great photos without plexiglass interference. Kelly, get in and make motor noises."

I didn't need a second invitation. When I sat down, my feet were about six inches from reaching the rudder pedals and I couldn't see out the windshield.

Dale laughed. "We don't let children fly."

In the back seat, there were extra cushions. With one in place and the seat adjusted, I sat just right. "This sure has a complete panel. Is he instrument rated?"

"I see he spent some big bucks on instrumentation. Even has a moving map GPS. Of course, the FAA still won't let us rely on them unless they are FAA certified."

"He must have expected to fly a lot."

"The GPS costs a fortune. Most pilots use them but have the backup standard instrumentation to meet all the regulations, which is what he has. I'm sure he flew IFR, with this kind of equipment."

I pushed on the pedals. Pulled back and pushed forward on the yoke and then turned full right and full left. Dale smiled as he watched me.

"Well, girl, what do you think?"

"You're the expert, but I like it."

"For the year, it's very good. The interior is in good condition. His log books are carefully maintained, all in a zippered folder. If he's been as careful with the plane as he has about his record keeping, I think this is a good plane."

I did some quick math in my brain. Maybe I could just write a check for the entire amount. "Would you ask your mechanic friend to go over it for me? Do you want a check to pay him in advance?"

"I'll take you home so you can get on with getting ready for work. This evening, I'll call the owner and tell him what we are up to and that you are interested."

I thanked Dale when he dropped me off. He seemed to be very pleased with himself. He also looked like he'd just showered instead of looking like he had just crawled out from under a rock.

Lynn was anxious to talk to me when I got to work. She was all smiles.

"Now I know what that funny expression was on your face when I left this morning. A big surprise awaited me. Dale and I went and looked at the plane. Great surprise!"

"I knew you'd be pleased. There is no one in the waiting room to be seen. Walk out with me."

Lynn stopped outside the door. "I had a long talk with Dale last night after I left here. He walked into the apartment with a beer in his hand. He'd been drinking on the way over. I laid it out straight that I was not interested in a drunk and if he didn't shape up I'd break off our relationship. I didn't say anything about you and Rob thinking he was drinking on the job, but I reminded him that one DUI would cost him his job."

"I'm glad you talked to him. He looked terrific today. Seemed happy. I appreciate his help with the airplane. I'm not very knowledgeable about the details of purchasing one."

"He really wanted to help you. I wasn't sure how he'd take my ultimatum. I have seen him close to violent before, though he's never touched me. He looked hurt and offended, walked over and poured the beer down the drain. He took my hand and sat us down on the couch side by side. Said when he was younger, drinking was a big problem for him. He said now he doesn't think it's a problem, he can stop any time, just enjoys it, but if I want him to stop or cut back, he will."

"Well, we can hope for the best and keep an eye on his behavior. If you see anything, you better say something right away."

"I'm heading home. We might go out to a movie tonight. Hope the ER is quiet."

Work was very quiet. In the morning, I slept till noon and then went down to my bank. After taking so little time off and working long hours since arriving in Alaska, I had saved almost enough to pay cash for the airplane. I talked to a loan officer, who encouraged me to pay about half and take a loan for the rest. That way, I would have a cushion for unforeseen expenses. It was a higher interest rate than I'd like, but it was still a good idea. I could pay it off rapidly with no penalty.

I drove down to the CAP office to see if anything was going on. The place looked deserted. I walked out into the large hangar housing two Beavers and the Cessna 310 we flew to McGrath. My footsteps on the cement floor echoed against the high steel roof. The lights were on. I flipped the switch off and turned to leave. I ran square into a tall man standing inches from me. On impact, I smelled his sweat and felt his body warmth.

Large hands grabbed my shoulders.

I screamed one of those startle screams that nearly caught in my throat. I knew immediately in the semidarkness who it was. He stood over me. I couldn't move.

Birdman.

"Dr. McKay, I didn't mean to scare you. My new sneakers are really quiet. I came down to sweep and clean up the place. Didn't hear you come in."

"John, my heart is still racing. I thought I was alone in this big place. Guess I'm jumpy today. Hope I didn't scare you."

He stared. "Me? Nothing bothers me except the voices. They're quiet now that I'm taking the medicine." His thoughts looked faraway. His eyes were not focusing on my face; he was staring through me. His face was void of expression and then, his head suddenly cocked as though he was listening intently to something I didn't hear.

"It's good you're taking the medicine." I had to get out of there. I lied, "I have to run. I'm meeting someone in a few minutes."

His voice was low, words slow and pleading. "Will you take me for a flight sometime?"

"Sure, John."

He droned on, no expression in his voice or face, "Sometimes I sit here with Leo in the radio room and listen to your voice on the radio when you're up flying."

I let the outside door slam so he'd know I'd left. My hands trembled as I tried to get my car key into the ignition.

John looked good, though drugged. I had nothing to be afraid of. I would have screamed no matter who it was behind me.

After an afternoon nap, I walked into a typical wild Saturday night. One of the nurses said, "Kelly, I hope you have your running shoes on. There are already three drunks lined up to be stitched. It's early enough that we might have the opportunity to see them again before the night is through if they go back out to party. At least no overdoses yet."

I ran from one room to the next for four hours, never quite catching up. There were always people waiting to be seen, sometimes six or eight at a time. Ambulances hauled people in and dropped them off, only to be called back out before they were finished with their paper work on the last one. Even Vic, who was typically a calm man, became exasperated. "Why don't these people use some moderation? They drink too much and get stupid." He headed off to clean up another suture room.

My charts to dictate were stacked high. By 3 a.m., I hadn't done one of them. The rooms were nearly full, but everyone had been evaluated. Most of them were waiting for labs or discharge orders. I was able to sit down for the first time all night. Vic placed a cup of coffee in front of me. "Made it myself. It's strong enough to keep you going for the rest of the shift."

"Thank you. I like strong coffee." I took a sip and opened my eyes wide.

"Vic, what is this? It's delicious."

"I brought my espresso maker with me tonight. It's a triple shot made with hazelnut coffee and real cream."

"It's delicious. Thank you."

"The others have already had one. You've been too busy. One doc, four nurses. Doesn't seem fair."

Before one chart was dictated, the scanner came alive, "Woman down, bleeding, assault victim."

The address was not far from the hospital. The next radio transmission for us was from the ambulance. "We are code 3 to your facility with an unresponsive woman with head and neck injuries. Intubated, no lines. We're two minutes out."

We met them at the door to help. The paramedic appeared stressed. He spilled out a rambling report as we wheeled her into a room and lifted her to an ER gurney. "Dr. McKay, she was gasping when we got to her, then she went out on me. I got the tube in, but it was tough. Had to use a smaller one than I thought she'd take." He showed me her neck. "You can see her neck is huge, there's a deep groove. Bruised, but with no bleeding. I think her trachea is fractured."

I examined her as he spoke. "She's been tachycardic in the 120s. Bleeding from her left thigh is from a jagged wound. We just slapped a pad on it. Haven't really looked at."

His partner added, "A patrol car saw her lying beside the road a few blocks away and called us. Nobody around. Didn't have time to get a line in. That's all we know."

While he was still talking, two nurses readied IV lines. They paged respiratory therapy to bring a ventilator and manage the airway. I looked her over following the simplistic ABC method: airway, breathing, circulation. Her airway was secure, with good placement of the tube. Breath sounds were equal on both sides, confirming the tube hadn't slid into the right mainstem bronchus or dislodged when we moved her. For circulation, she had a strong pulse with a heart rate of 110.

Medics helped slice off her clothes and turned her to check her back. Her pupils were reactive, and she was breathing some on her own. Her exam showed no other marks except a jagged deep laceration in her lateral thigh.

Police came in after finding her identification and checking out her residence. A neighbor told them she worked as a night stocker at a local grocery.

I summarized my findings to the police. "So, we have a woman who's been assaulted. Her vital signs are stable, but she appears to have anoxic brain injury from her airway injury. With all the subcutaneous air in her neck and the trouble intubating, her trachea is damaged. She was probably choked with a wire, a garrote."

Vic stood by, "What do you want next, Doc? Urine drug screen? Head CT scan?"

I fired back. "Both. Add a comprehensive chemistry panel, pregnancy test, CBC, cross-table cervical spine X-ray, and put her in a hard-collar. Pile warm blankets on her and give her warmed IV fluids at a rate of 150 milliliters per hour. Foley catheter, too. Eventually, she needs a tetanus immunization, and I'll need a suture tray with supplies for a two-layer closure."

After the rapid exam and initiation of orders, I started over, beginning with her head, and performed a detailed examination. I found no swelling of her scalp. Her ears and mouth were negative too. Around her eyes, tiny, ruptured blood vessels called petechiae showed changes from the strangulation. Her carotid artery pulsation felt normal, in spite of the swollen, bruised neck. Her hard-working hands were calloused and had manicured nails. A couple of the nails were broken, and one fingertip was sliced off and bleeding.

Detectives arrived. The policemen who had found her filled them in on the crime scene details. After taking photos of her injuries, they quickly did the evidence collection. Their primary interest was in nail scrapings and, of course, having me perform a rape exam. A rape exam could take a couple hours when dealing with emotional cases, but in her comatose state it would be much faster.

The scan showed no brain injury, no bleeding, and no skull fracture but confirmed tracheal injury with extensive soft tissue air. No blood collections. Her neck vertebrae showed no fractures.

We followed the rape collection protocol in detail, not wanting to miss anything. I swabbed all the appropriate places, including inside her vagina. Saliva and hair samples completed our specimen collection. The chain of evidence was completed when I signed and sealed the box and handed it to the detectives without it ever being out of our sight.

I requested a bed for her in ICU. The neurosurgeon on call was not impressed. "Doesn't sound surgical to me, Kelly. Why don't you just call someone to manage her vent? I'll consult regarding her head. She might need surgery on her neck. If there's much anoxic downtime, we'll see brain swelling within the next couple hours. If that happens, then I'll come in and do a bolt to measure brain pressures and help with her management. What do you think?"

"Well, I'll see what I can do. I see your point. I called you first because it appears that her primary problem is anoxic brain injury. Based on her presentation, I think she'll need intracranial pressure monitoring. Would you be sure to see her first thing in the morning? Sooner, if they call?"

"Sure. Order another CT scan of her head in three hours. Have them call me before that if there is any change in her condition."

I asked the secretary to call another sleeping surgeon. It's kind of like waking a sleeping dog. I like to be at least the second person to talk to them—it gives time for the angry outbursts to dissipate.

I used my most cheerful voice, hoping it would calm him and not incite profanity. "Hi, Peter, it's four a.m. and way too early for anyone to be up. I have a problem in the ER and need some advice."

First a deep sigh, then, "Whatcha got?"

"A young woman with an unusual injury, garrote-type assault with tracheal injury. Her neck is grossly swollen due to air in the tissues, and she has anoxic brain injury. I called you because I'm concerned about a vascular injury. I already talked to neurosurgery. She may need a pressure bolt."

"I'm awake now, Kelly. I'll come right in. Call the radiologist. We need to do stat vascular studies of her neck to be sure there's no dissection. Has her neck been enlarging since you got her intubated?"

"No. She hasn't changed. I can feel her carotid pulses."

"Just keep doing neuros. Watch her pupils. If she dissects or occludes a carotid, she'll go down fast. It will take me about fifteen minutes to get there."

"Thanks so much. I'll suture her leg laceration while you're en route."

Nurses had anesthetized and irrigated the laceration. All I had to do was stitch. The wound was about five inches long, into muscle. It required a two-layer closure, a deep row of absorbable stitches followed by skin sutures. The nurse who came in to dress it commented, "Funny-looking injury. Looks like an 'M.'"

Just as she was being wheeled to Radiology the police entered with an overweight middle-aged man with long blond hair and hands cuffed behind his back. My first thought was a probable DUI and that they needed a legal blood alcohol draw.

Vic took one look and motioned them into the lockdown room.

They walked past and I realized the man was wearing a woman's wig. He looked back suspiciously and struggled to free his hands as they marched him down the hall. His tooled leather belt told me his name, *Butch*.

One of the officers took me aside. "Neighbors called 9-1-1 after he discharged his rifle in the back yard. He lives out at the edge of town. They thought he might be firing at a bear, but he wouldn't answer the phone, so they got worried."

The second officer said, "We're always concerned about what we might find and are wary any time a "shots fired" call comes in. At the door, we identified ourselves and he opened the door a crack. After he verified we were police, he invited us right in."

The patient listened to the information they were giving me. He added to the narrative. "The cops made it just in time. They were closing in on me, so I threw a blanket over the television set to keep them from watching me."

I walked closer to Butch. "Thanks for telling us what was happening."

The man looked at me through blond strands and wiped his sweaty forehead.

The first officer said, "He hasn't given us any trouble. His home is barricaded with furniture. He had a chair against the wall and had loaded guns, with stacks of ammo on the table. He thinks somebody's after him. He insisted on wearing his wig as a disguise."

His stringy hair tangled in his unshaven gray stubble. A grimy T-shirt failed to cover his hanging-over belly. "Doctor, I don't *think* they're after me, I *know* they're after me."

One of the officers said, "So, how about taking off that stupid wig? You're safe here with us and talking to the doctor."

Butch adjusted his wig. "I'm not talkin' anymore. I ain't tellin' you nothin.'"

The cop reached for the wig. "You better start talking or we're taking you to jail."

Not wanting to rile the disturbed man, I stopped the officer from taking the wig. "Hello, Butch, I'm Dr. McKay. I'll take care of you. You look scared tonight. What are you afraid of?"

He slowly looked up at me with eyes like a tired, beaten dog. "Who told you my name?"

"I read your name on that tooled belt you're wearing. Did you make that yourself?"

"Rose gave it to me."

"Who's Rose?"

"Rose is my wife. I really miss her. After she moved out, things just went to hell. I've heard voices before, but they've been after me constantly since she left. I haven't slept a wink in two weeks. She'll tell you about the voices. I was trying to make it without medication because it costs too much, but I started drinking to stop the voices. The voices go away when I sleep. Now, I just can't get to sleep."

He glanced over his shoulder and scanned the room. "If the cops will stay and protect us, I'll talk to you some more."

They agreed and hung out in the doorway.

Butch began. "My name is Alexander Johnson. My mom named me a big fancy name 'cause Johnson is so common, but I've been Butch all my life. When I was little, I called myself Zander. Everybody ended up calling me Butch."

I sat beside him and just let him talk.

"I've heard voices since I was a kid. I thought everybody did till I was a teenager. Rose is the only one that has ever treated me right. She has voices, too. She understands. She said she loved me even though I was paranoid as hell, but she couldn't take the drinking. She's been gone for days. I think she's at her mother's."

He put his head down, the wig hanging forward into his lap. He sobbed.

"Butch, wouldn't Rose want you to get well? You need to take your medicine. Do you know what medicine you are supposed to take?"

"They know me at the psycho hospital. They'll know. I like it there. Can I go there till I'm not scared anymore?"

I called the Alaska Psychiatric Institute. They gave me his last medication list and agreed to admit him. I ordered a starting dose of his meds from the pharmacy and went back with the first dose. "Butch, the nurse at API told me your medicine. I have it here. Take this right away so it will start working. I need to listen to your heart and lungs and check you over to be sure you're all right before the police give you a ride next door."

Butch took his antipsychotic medication. "Tomorrow, can I call Rose?"

"That sounds reasonable. Why don't you ask when you get to API?"

Butch was our last patient of the night.

When the day shift arrived, I still had two hours of dictation to complete.

Chapter 15 Trouble

Lynn was still sleeping when I went to bed. I had no intention of sleeping more than four hours because I was off for a couple of days. I stuffed earplugs in and lay down. The phone rang and rang. I assumed Lynn would answer it, but the ringing continued. I finally rolled over and picked it up. "Hello."

A deep muffled male voice said, "Kelly, is that you?"

"Yes."

"Kelly, are you tired after working so hard?"

"Who is this?"

"Don't work too hard." Dial tone.

I didn't recognize the voice and was angry about the rude awakening.

I prowled around the apartment, finding Lynn gone and a note saying she was shopping and would meet Dale for lunch.

Who had called to harass me? Brett Warren? It didn't sound like him. He wouldn't dare show his face.

I went back to bed. Lying in my darkened bedroom, exhausted, churning thoughts kept me awake for a long time.

The doorbell, sounds of pounding, and someone rattling the door jarred my tired brain awake again. Green numbers on the digital clock glowed 12:20. The pounding continued.

Dressed in sweats, I went to the door, furious, and jerked it open. "What the hell do you want?"

Dumb move. I should have used the peek hole.

There stood my former drug addict boyfriend, Brett Warren.

I grabbed the door to close it.

He kicked his foot forward, blocking the door. His tremulous hand touched my arm. "Kelly, I won't hurt you. You aren't being very friendly."

"How did you find me?"

"I went to the hospital to ask for you. I followed you home. It took a while to get up the courage to come here. I need help. I saw Lynn leave. So, you're roommates?"

I said nothing, not quite sure what to do to get rid of him.

"Can I come in? I screwed up big time. I couldn't hack the stupid chemical dependency program. They're assholes. Not a clue what it's really like to have a drug problem. I need to get off the shit and stay off. They wanted to put me in a methadone program. I can't do surgery on methadone. Can I please come in, Kelly? I won't hurt you."

"Brett, I'm afraid of you. I'm afraid with you blocking the door open. I might talk to you some time when there is someone else here, when Lynn is with me. I've been up all night. I'm tired. I need to sleep. Please leave."

"Kelly, I don't want to leave. I don't have any place to go. My folks bought me a ticket up here."

"So, what are you doing? Do you have drug money?"

"No. I was hoping you'd help me out just this once with a place to stay and some cash."

"Brett, I'm no fool. I was once, but never again. You're on your own. If you need help, go to the ER and ask for directions to the CD program. Check yourself in."

He looked down at his foot, dejected. He moved back, tense and shaky, in withdrawal. He put his hands in his pockets. "Kelly, I had to see you. I loved you. I still do. I'm sorry I bothered you."

"Did you call about two hours ago?"

He shook his head and shuffled away.

I waited a minute and then looked down the street. He was walking slowly toward the hospital.

I double-locked the front door. This time, it was *my* hand that was shaking.

I checked the deck door. Locked.

Those locks are notoriously poorly made, so I blocked any door movement with a stick on the bottom in the travel groove. Feeling safe, I returned to bed, but I was still awake when Lynn and Dale came in.

I opened my door and found them locked in a kiss.

After they realized they had company, I received a warm greeting. "Oh, Kel, the most wonderful thing has happened. We're celebrating. Dale asked me to marry him, and I said yes!"

I smelled liquor, which sent a negative stabbing jolt that I tried to cover. "Wow! Congratulations! That is quite a plunge. Are you sure you're ready?"

Dale responded. "We're ready, really ready. We're talking about having an outdoor wedding. Really outdoor. On a mountaintop somewhere."

I gave them hugs. "That's great. I'm happy for you."

They clung to each other, hopefully not for support. "So, what did you celebrate with?"

"Rusty nails. We each had two," Lynn slurred.

"Scotch and Drambuie. It's a little heavy for lunch, but hell, we're celebrating."

"This is the second shock I've had already this afternoon. This one is much, much better than the first."

Lynn asked, "What else?"

"Brett Warren was here."

"I knew we'd be seeing him. What did he want?"

"A place to live, money, companionship."

"He has balls."

"He was twitchy. I think he's in withdrawal. I was so sleepy I opened the door without looking." I explained what happened. "He tried to sweet-talk me."

"God, Kelly, that was dumb of you to open the door. Then what? How did you get him to leave?"

"I said no to all his requests. I told him to go to the ER and get a referral to a drug program. He gave me a 'how could you' hang-dog look and dejectedly left. I haven't been able to get back to sleep, so I might as well stay up."

"How did he know we lived here?"

"He followed me home this morning. I had a creepy feeling but saw nothing suspicious. I went to bed, and a call awakened me after noon. Don't know who it was for sure, but he called me by name. I assume it was Brett. He watched you leave the apartment."

Lynn opened her bedroom door. "I need to sleep. We're going to nap."

"I'm going out to Merrill to set up some flight instructions. Dale, did the mechanic check out the plane yet?"

"He called this morning. Compression checks are good. Needs no repairs." Dale reached in his shirt pocket and pulled out a spiral notebook. "Here, let me write down the owner's name and phone for you. Set up a time to meet him at your bank."

They disappeared into Lynn's bedroom and closed the door.

Chapter 16 Flying

By the end of the productive morning, I had talked to the mechanic, the bank, and the plane owner. A few signed papers, and it was mine! I made an appointment to meet the instructor Dale had recommended at Peggy's restaurant, and after talking with him on the phone, I was scheduled for the first lesson in my own plane. The weather had me concerned. It was sunny but with strong winds and low clouds rolling in off Cook Inlet. I knew two things for sure: a crosswind is not good flying weather, and after such disrupted sleep, I wasn't at my best.

I was very excited to finally have accomplished another long-term goal. I'd finished medical training, completed the Boards, had a stable job, and, finally, I owned a plane! I had no one to share the good news with except Lynn. If I called my sister and mother in Minnesota, neither would be very happy because of our family history.

The aircraft manual kept me company while I waited for the instructor. A tall, skinny man wearing jeans and a flannel plaid shirt walked in and surveyed the patrons. He was about fifty, with nearly white short hair and a trimmed gray beard. He hesitantly asked, "You Doc McKay?"

I stood up and shook Tab's outstretched hand. I liked the deep smile wrinkles crinkling around his dark eyes.

The waitress followed him. "The usual?"

He nodded. "You want a refill on your coffee, Dr. McKay?"

She returned with tea for him and a refill for me.

"So, you want to get some more taildragger time?"

"I own an airplane I'm not authorized to fly it. Sounds pretty dumb."

"It's not dumb. You just need time in it."

"Most of my flying has been with tricycle gear. On landing, taildraggers feel squirrelly."

"We call them 'training wheels.' Once you set 'em down, they track straight and stable. Not so with a taildragger. You have to stay on it and fly till you park it. It is different than what you are used to, so it feels unstable."

After looking at my flight log, license, and medical, he reviewed some flying characteristics with me. He drew cute little airplane pictures on napkins with arrows for wind. "Everyone worries about ground-looping in crosswinds. Today is a good day to take you up. We can fly one runway and do basics with the wind straight down the runway. Then we'll do direct crosswind work off the other runway."

That generated immediate fear in my heart. Would we crash my brand-new airplane on my first flight?

Tab continued, "I ground-looped my Maule a couple years ago. Thought I had it made. Reached for something, and it left the runway in a flash. When that happened, I had a thousand hours in taildraggers from my crop-dusting days. I haven't lived it down. Thought I might as well tell you about it 'cause somebody else will if I don't."

"Dale didn't mention it."

"He was being kind."

I wanted Tab to get right to the specifics, so I opened the instruction manual to "Wheel Landings." "Talk to me about these."

"Some instructors will tell you to do wheel landings. I don't like 'em. Three pointers will take you through anything. I have to teach you wheel landings because the FAA, in their wisdom, deems it necessary. I'll demonstrate and talk you through some. It's easier than sitting at a table talking about it."

In the airplane, he spoke in a comforting tone. "You won't ground-loop and crack it up unless you aren't paying attention. With the wind blowing this strong, you have to keep the ailerons cranked into the wind until the last minute before touching down. Then once you are down, crank it in again. The wind against the wings will hold you down if you have the ailerons in the correct position. If you don't, the wind will get under that wing and the lift will whip it right around and meet you coming." He demonstrated the techniques he had discussed.

I nodded, understanding what he meant.

He emphasized, "You want to do a three-point landing and, once you're down, keep it down. Be on it all the time. Keep the plane in the center of the runway. Do lots of little corrections. If you get on the brakes too much when you're going fast, watch out for the pucker brush. You'll turn fast, exit the runway, and dip a wing in the dirt in one swift move."

We spent close to the first hour just "flyin' like a crop duster." Using the runway as an imaginary field to be sprayed, we flew a few feet off the ground. The wind tried to blow us off course. I got better and better at keeping it right down the centerline. As soon as I had accomplished that, he added landings.

I was tense but found I could do it. After about a dozen landings, my legs were Jell-O and I wanted to quit. Then he said, "It's time to do wheel landings."

My body begged to go home, but I had learned so much in one day that I couldn't bear to quit.

He demonstrated a wheel landing on the favorable runway without the crosswind to distract me. "Once you touch down, push forward on the stick slightly to keep it on the runway. Maintain the forward stick to keep the tail up as long as possible."

When he did it, it seemed fun, and it gave better visibility of the runway ahead. The first landing I did was horrible, though, like a bucking bronco. I almost dinged the prop on the runway, and he had to take over the controls.

"I don't like this. It seems unnatural. Pushing forward made me feel like it would go right over on the prop."

He assured me it was very unlikely because of the way the plane was designed and rigged. "When the tail stops flying, it will settle to the runway and you'll be back to three points."

Taxiing back to the ramp was a challenge for me too. I found myself using the brakes a lot just to maintain control and turn in the strong wind.

Tab said, "Don't worry about the brakes. We use them more in taildraggers because they don't maneuver on the ground like tricycles. You've got the hang of it, Doc. The winds today were a perfect introduction."

"I appreciate your calmness. My other instructors were twitchy. Hope I didn't frighten you."

"You didn't. You know why they call me Tab, don't you? Didn't Dale tell you? It actually stands for 'turn and bank.' I took up aerobatics a few years ago. A couple more hours and I'll sign you off. Then, you need to start thinking about flying inverted. It's a kick in the pants." He waved as he strode off to a double-cab pickup with a big tail-wagging dog in the back seat.

I got home and reached for the phone to call Dale to thank him for telling me about Tab. It rang loudly just as my hand touched it. I answered in a happy voice.

On the other end, nothing. Then heavy breathing, faster and faster, as if orgasmic. I slammed the receiver down and locked the doors.

Later, I called Dale. I told him I had gotten an obscene phone call. He laughed. "Some guy gettin' his nuts off at your expense. He must like you."

"It makes me mad. I don't feel safe in my own house. I really called to tell you how much I liked Tab. He's an excellent pilot and instructor. A couple of hours with him made me realize how little I know about flying, real flying. He's so calm."

"I knew you'd like his style."

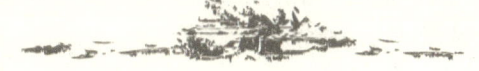

The month of May brought longer hours of daylight but frost at night. The Chugach Range remained white on the higher elevations. After I got my endorsement, I took Lynn flying. We went to Wasilla to visit Ed and Lucille. They had tiny puppies, three weeks old.

"Pick one out, Kelly. When it gets big enough you can take it home. Teach it to go flying while it's young." Ed looked in my eyes. "You should get one with blue eyes like yours."

"Get one, Kelly. Dale and I will help you take care of it." Lynn held a tiny dog. "It's so adorable."

"I'm afraid to hold one. I already want one, Ed. Right now, it wouldn't be fair to get one. I'm gone thirteen to fourteen hours a day. Lynn, you and Dale work the same kind of hours I do. I want one when I'm not working so much."

"After Dale and I get married, we'll have a house with a yard. Then, maybe we can get two and share dog sitting."

Ed beamed like a new father. "Just let me know when."

We flew back toward Anchorage. Lynn looked down along our flight path. "I think we're over the Eagle River. If you follow the river, you can hike from here up to Raven Glacier and over Crow Creek Pass to the other side."

I circled lower. "I see some hikers."

"Last summer, I went to Crow Creek Pass from the south side with one of the nurses. It's a beautiful hike. You just go to the ski area turnoff, then go left. Let's do an overnight."

"When are we off together again?"

"Dale works over Memorial Day, but I'm off. I don't want to hang around home on a three-day weekend."

I climbed higher to the summit. "I'll check my schedule when we get home."

"There is a Forest Service cabin just over the summit. Let's see if we can find it."

I banked and turned in the direction she pointed. "There is a little structure surrounded by snow. Maybe we should wait till later in the summer."

We looked down on the small cabin in the snow. Below, a trail with switchbacks left the snow and descended steeply among large boulders and exposed terrain. The zig-zag trail disappeared into the trees.

Lynn sounded enthused. "It's not bad. It's a very well-traveled, popular hike. If it isn't already reserved, we could rent the cabin. Otherwise, just go up and down in one day. It's not a long hike, only three thousand feet in three miles and you're at the summit."

Chapter 17 A Mountain Hike

Lynn, wrapped up in an oversized yellow polar fleece jacket, put her baseball hat on backwards, fastened her seat belt, and scrunched down for the drive to the Crow Creek Pass trailhead. "I'm ready to roll."

We sped south in my Subaru, leaving Anchorage just an image in the rearview mirror. Cool, fresh air washed through the open windows, blowing my hair in swirls. "It's so good to be out of that ER commotion and into this beautiful country. It feels good to be underway, a reprieve. We've been working too much."

"Kelly, what you really mean is you're leaving behind the uneasiness of knowing Brett is in town. He can't follow us to Crow Creek. You've acted more on edge since he arrived."

"I don't think he'd hurt me. He saved my life. But I don't trust him, and on drugs, even less. I'll try to forget about him and pay attention to my driving. I love to drive. I would rather drive than ride, except maybe in your 928." I rambled on. "When I was ten, my grandfather taught me to drive a grain truck along the fields on his farm during harvest. I was so short I could only reach the pedals with blocks on them and pillows behind my back. Kind of like I fly airplanes now."

Lynn laughed, "Yeah, you're older, but you haven't grown much."

"Grandpa told me I was a wonderful driver, best he ever had."

The route along Turnagain Arm took us along narrow tidal waters on one side and mountainous terrain on the other. Rimmed by the mountains ahead and looking southward across the water, the views were like picture postcards.

Lynn looked relaxed and pensive. Suddenly she sat up straight. "Kelly, pull over."

I braked abruptly and headed for the shoulder. "What's wrong?"

"I'm sorry. It's not an emergency. I just meant park where you can. There's a turnoff ahead. I have to see why the cars are stopped. Maybe there's a wild animal near the road."

I pulled off the highway just past McHugh Creek at Beluga Point. On the opposite side of the road, a line of parked cars and tourists stood with their cameras pointed up the slope away from the water.

We walked across the highway to join them and saw a dozen mountain goats, some with little babies, grazing and looking down at the tourists. I took many photos before we walked back across the highway, across the railroad tracks, and down a rocky embankment to the tidal flats.

Lynn pointed. "See that warning sign not to walk out onto the flats because of quicksand and rapid incoming tides? It's a terrible hazard that people don't seem to recognize. Last summer a guy walked out there and mired down. His friends couldn't get him out before the tide came in and drowned him."

"That's ugly. What a way to die."

"I like walking the shore at low tide. You have to be sure you stay along the shore. I've seen a dozen eagles down there near the waterline. They are amazing to watch."

Looking east, my eyes followed the shoreline. There were no eagles today. Instead, near us, seagulls fought for tasty morsels exposed by the low tide. They pecked and rummaged over food they found in the smelly green plant life.

Looking due west, the water stretched forever.

Lynn pointed up a mountain slope. "We are headed up there."

I followed her hand. The coastal mountains rose sharply, with a dense fog layer obscuring the lower slopes.

"We have to stop at the Birdhouse. It's a popular local landmark and worth stopping for. Let's go."

A man-sized neon parrot holding a champagne glass hung drunkenly from the front of a ramshackle building. I didn't see the sign until we got so close that I had to brake hard and crank into the driveway. We stopped in a cloud of dust next to a tour bus and trooped along a railing and boardwalk to the entrance, where there was a line of people. "This looks like a place Duke Bradshaw could ride over to on his horse and tie it up outside while he was in drinking a beer."

"It does have a Western feel. I miss Duke. I hope he and Betsy are doing well on their ranch in Montana. It's too bad we couldn't attend the wedding last fall because we were the newcomers and all the guys wanted time off to hunt."

"When we were in Seattle, I talked to one of our Harbor Medical Center friends who attended." Lynn stepped inside the bar and waited for her eyes to adjust in the darkness and then continued. "The wedding party was a blast. They put people up in the bunkhouse. Duke is working part-time as a radiologist."

"I could fly us down for a visit when things settle down here."

Lynn agreed "Let's do it in the early fall before all the hunters decide they have to make us work nonstop again." She led the way inside the tilted log cabin.

I ducked my head to enter through the low frame doorway. The interior was very dark and smelled pleasantly of the wood chips scattered on the floor in a thick, soft carpet. The darkness inside was a marked contrast to the morning sun.

As my vision adjusted, I saw walls and a low ceiling completely papered with business cards of previous patrons. It was standing room only until the bus driver loomed in the doorway. He held his arm high and pointed at his watch. The crowd vanished with him.

Lynn chose seating at the bar. We sat on stools that were nothing more than logs standing on end.

I whispered, "This is not the sort of place your mother would enter. Do you plan to bring her here for shock value when she comes to visit?"

"You bet. That's why I brought you here. I think it's part of the Alaskan experience—dirt floors, wood shavings, and wonderful people. The bartenders are fun. Mother would like meeting them because it would give her a real story for her prissy friends."

The ancient bar, marred with carved initials and hearts, angled at about a 20-degree downhill slant toward the wall. The bartender waited to take our order as we squinted to make out details in the darkness. When my eyes finally adjusted, I saw him smiling, maybe laughing at us.

He was a people watcher, enjoying the expressions of disbelief on his customers.

Lynn explained, "Someone told me the ground shifted in the 1964 earthquake and they just left the bar this way. You either have to hang onto your drink or park it against the little bumpers glued to the surface."

My eyes fixated on the end of the bar where a large jar of boiled eggs sat with a sign reading *Boneless Chicken Dinners two for fifty cents, three for a dollar.*

Pieces of clothing dangled over the bar among the business cards. A dusty rubber chicken, missing a leg, hung by its neck.

I ordered whiskey with diet 7-Up. Lynn ordered rum and diet Coke.

The bartender's eyes twinkled. "How about a pickle to go with your low-calorie drinks? Makes a nice breakfast. Pickles are low calorie." The label on the pickle jar suggested they were *very hot* pepper pickles.

We shook our heads no.

He set up the drinks. "Have you ladies seen any ptarmigan in your travels?"

I looked at Lynn. "I'm not sure I'd know one if I saw one."

She shook her head. "I've never seen one."

The bartender rummaged beneath the bar and came up with a brass horn that looked like a miniature French horn with a few unusual corkscrew turns. "Blow on this and look out the window. A ptarmigan usually shows up."

I envisioned a new form of life appearing when I blew.

His little smirk and bright eyes made me wary.

I blew hard. A fine spray of white powder filled the air.

Everyone at the bar laughed.

The bartender explained, "Ptarmigan are very difficult to see and identify. In fact, the word is difficult to spell, so difficult to spell that the citizens of Chicken, Alaska, finally settled on Chicken because no one could spell ptarmigan."

We both laughed, although I wasn't sure how much of it was a joke. But, whatever the joke, it was certainly on us.

A young woman sat down at the bar across from us and peered into the dingy room. She pulled out a cigarette and ordered a beer.

The bartender quickly came to her assistance and lit the cigarette with the biggest lighter I'd ever seen. It was the size of a large box of cereal and almost set fire to the extra-large red bra that hung over the woman's head.

A grimy-looking male of about twenty-five slid onto the barstool next to the woman and ordered a tap beer. He cocked his head to the side as if listening to her and lit a cigarette.

She said nothing and stared down into her drink.

Smoke from his cigarette and hers intermingled in a sunbeam that found its way across the bar from a crack in the shuttered window behind us.

The bartender took a deep breath and lurched toward the man. Cold eye contact penetrated the man's stare. He turned away from the woman. A scar crossed his right eyebrow and dived into his cheek. Green serpents wrapped both his arms, and when he drank from his glass, the tattoos gave the illusion that the serpents were feeding him.

I elbowed Lynn and whispered. "Let's get the heck out of here. He's giving me the creeps."

We left our drinks behind. Lynn got in the car. "I didn't really want a drink but thought you should see the place. Wasn't it great?"

"It's certainly unique. How is Dale doing with his drinking?"

"Now don't spoil our trip by bugging me about him. He has a beer now and then, but he's cut way back. It's not a problem, Kelly, so lay off."

"I felt uncomfortable asking but felt I had to. I haven't seen any evidence of his drinking, but I believe if Rob smells anything on him at work, he'll blow the whistle. Dale will be drug-tested on the spot. It's not something trivial."

Lynn interrupted me by reading aloud a sign: "Erickson Gold Mine, Visitors Welcome. Have you ever panned for gold, Kelly?"

"No. I want to come back here sometime and try it. One of those things I have to do while I'm in Alaska."

"It might be fun to find a big nugget, but I'd rather stop at a jewelry store than slop around in dirt for a few flecks of gold. I hate to admit it, but I am like my mother in some ways."

We turned at the Alyeska Ski Area Road onto a winding narrow road to the Crow Creek Pass parking lot. A few miles up the bumpy road, we reached the trailhead, which was surrounded by trees.

There were three parked cars and no people in sight.

The trail disappeared into the fog.

Lynn and I had packed great food, including steaks and a bottle of red wine. We hoisted frame packs with sleeping bags and pads strapped on, and we carried enough water for the overnight trip. She snapped a canister of pepper spray onto her pack. "I feel dumb carrying pepper spray."

I took my pepper spray out of my frame pack and attached it to my belt. "I don't think there are any bears for miles around unless they're two-legged ones, but I feel more secure bringing it."

After an hour of steady hiking in dense fog, I looked around and said sarcastically, "Isn't the scenery great?"

"We'll be out of this soon. Just wait."

After more altitude gain that left me panting, we left wisps of fog and entered blinding sun. The difference from damp gloom to warmth was shocking. The view above the layer ended at the horizon.

"I told you, Kelly. What do you think?"

I sat on a large boulder and looked around. "This is amazing. Like flying above the clouds. I've popped through a fog layer into the sun flying, but never before when hiking."

The steep trail turned into the switchbacks we had seen from the air. Fist-sized rocks strewn along the trail made it treacherous and easy to turn an ankle. "There is much less snow than when I flew us over. Do think the cabin is still in the snow?"

She looked toward the summit. "I think we'll find snow up there."

The switchbacks continued to a high ridge near the summit. We had already covered some of the steepest terrain, not the least bit frightening or dangerous but not a trail one would want to run on because of the rocks strewn about. Other than a whistle from a marmot or a squawk of a jay, the silence was broken only by our breathing and trudging noises.

We reached the snowline and decided to rest on a large sun-warmed rock surrounded by icy melting snow. From there, we surveyed the world below as we ate our lunch of trail mix, French bread, cheese, and water.

To get to the cabin, we stayed on a narrow trail consisting of kick-steps left in the snow by others, now an icy path. It was steep enough that a fall would send us skidding like an out-of-control toboggan to the melt-line and onto the rocks. I slowed, but Lynn climbed without effort.

Once at the cabin, we dumped our packs and hiked the steeper snowy trail to the summit. Over the ridge, we looked down on the world toward Eagle River. Raven Glacier loomed blue and cold, hanging like a waterfall. Ahead, down a gentle incline, a large silver-gray object stuck out from the melting snow, part of crashed airplane fuselage. It had been stripped of its radios, instruments, and many parts, but a recognizable skeleton remained.

"They've lost a lot of planes up here in Alaska." I felt a shiver.

Lynn looked around. "I hear voices."

I listened and heard nothing. "Seeing this crash site gives me the creeps. Maybe they are voices of ghosts from the crash."

"I don't believe in ghosts and neither do you. Let's go to the cabin and start dinner. We can watch the sun over Cook Inlet."

I started back down the path, talking. "In Seattle, I used to like sunrise the best, but since coming to Alaska, I switched to watching sunsets. When I first got here, I went to tourist shops. I looked at hand-painted gold pans with their scenes and skies in such bright hues, they looked surreal. I knew they couldn't possibly exist. I was wrong."

Lynn laughed. "Gold pans don't lie. You have to experience a few sunsets to believe the colors."

"The sun doesn't really set in the summer. From up here, even this early, if we have clear skies tonight, just with the moonlight I bet we can see the horizon. You can see forever."

It was after six when we finally unrolled our sleeping bags in the loft. There was other sleeping space on the lower level, but the view was best from up high.

We cooked on our tiny white-gas Svea stoves set up on flat rocks. Our steaks sizzled. We lounged on boulders, admiring the world below, and sipped wine from stemmed plastic glasses.

We heard voices coming from behind the cabin while we were devouring the steaks. I checked for my pepper spray.

Two rugged college-age guys rounded the corner, smiling. "Are we just in time for dinner? Gosh, it smells good. Like hamburgers grilled outside at a ski area."

"The tall gangly tanned one jokingly asked, "What are you serving?"

"Steak and wine. You're welcome to join us, but we don't have enough to feed you."

His friend said, "He was kidding. We have food. Heck, we even have wine but don't have fancy glasses like yours."

They removed heavy packs and began unloading cooking utensils, food, and stoves. Their freeze-dried food needed water and smelled almost as good cooking as our steak. The four of us laughed, toasted, and talked well into the night.

At midnight, the dark sky was alive with stars. We just kept talking. They had just come from Eagle River across Crow Creek Pass from the north side. Twenty-eight miles and three river crossings at flood stage from the spring melt—not for the faint of heart. They looked very tired.

They didn't look or act like violent people. I hated being suspicious about everyone, but with Brett Warren back in town and that ugly phone call, I felt uneasy.

After the wine was gone, the talking slowed. They asked if we minded if they stayed for the night, outside the cabin, of course. They seemed so nice and genuine. I was ready to tell them they could sleep inside on the lower level. It was cold at this higher altitude.

Lynn elbowed me in the ribs to shut up.

They spread their sleeping bags out of the wind near the cabin.

Lynn slept.

I lay snuggled in my sleeping bag, looking at the night sky through the open window.

Slow breathing and an occasional snore penetrated the mountain silence. I closed my eyes, glad to be safe.

In the distance, a strange wail drifted to my nest in the loft.

I remained awake, listening to the mountain noises. The wind occasionally shook the cabin. There were no panes in the windows, so the wind blew straight through the loft.

I was startled by another wail in the distance and was glad we were on the upper level.

Maybe it was a marmot.

Chapter 18 Homicide

Lynn and I awakened to find the hikers gone. They left a thank-you note written on the cardboard from a food container. Our hot breakfast of reconstituted eggs and soy bacon was not as tasty as our evening meal, but we were hungry, and it tasted great.

A layer of clouds wrapped the lower mountainside and trail far below us. The sky above remained clear. Hiking downhill, our expansive view of the mountainside revealed historical evidence of human activity. Remnants of a water conduit and a collection of man-made items strewn about half a block off the trail caught my eye. "Lynn, let's take a closer look."

She veered off immediately, going fast enough to make me pant keeping up.

The debris turned out to be the remnants of some sort of mining site, with a few recognizable rusting cans and skeletal bed springs. I picked up a broken pipe along a steep rocky slope that might have been part of a water conduit. "I wonder if they found much gold?"

"Probably not since it's abandoned, but there must be some with the Erickson Gold Mine nearby and still active."

Back on the trail, we passed a young couple hiking up with a boy about five years old who skipped along with a white-haired elderly man. Grandpa didn't look tired going uphill, yet we were sweating going downhill. I asked him, "How can you look so good on this strenuous hike?"

He ruffled the boy's red hair. "I've been walking at least three miles a day since I retired twenty years ago. Besides I have to keep up with my grandson."

When I glanced back at them later, grandpa and grandson were having a snowball fight, their contrasting hair shining in the sun.

We reached the tree line, where clouds carried inland by a sea breeze off Turnagain Arm obscured the sun, and we hiked down into a dark, misty area. It felt cool now that we were out of the sun on the open terrain. Lynn was ahead of me. We were almost back to the parking lot when I heard a chilling gasp, followed by a scream and running footsteps.

I reached for my bear spray.

Lynn ran into me with such force that I lost my footing, and we both fell.

She pushed me down, trying to get back to her feet.

Lynn looked pale and pointed to the ground ahead.

We got to our feet, and I saw a stiff blue foot with red-painted toenails protruding from beneath some bushes.

We stood perfectly still, holding our breath.

I heard my own heart pounding and Lynn's stilted breathing.

I armed the pepper spray, not knowing what good it would do or what to expect. I scanned ahead and behind. I saw nothing.

Silence

Fog clung to the trees around the body.

I stepped closer to look at the young female's skin, mottled with the unmistakable blotches of death.

The dependent parts of her body were purple.

Her ripped bra exposed a breast with a ring through the nipple.

A red rose tattoo extended above the ring.

Her purple thong underwear nearly matched the color of the fireweed plant blooming beside her bony hip.

A slightly different hue of purple colored her distorted face and neck.

I heard the high-pitched buzz of a few flies that were landing periodically and then taking flight again, collecting on the blood crusting around her neck and leg. My voice sounded loud. "There's no rank odor. She hasn't been here long."

Lynn hadn't moved. "Do you think she was there on our way up?"

"Maybe. We might not have seen her in the fog."

Lynn brushed past me. "Let's get out of here."

We ran the rest of the way through the fog. I tripped once and grabbed Lynn's arm. She gasped and ran faster. Finally, we reached the opening of the parking lot, empty except for two cars and an old green van. We threw our backpacks into the car, jumped in, and slammed and locked all the doors.

Lynn was breathing hard, and I was shaking so much, we just sat there for a few minutes. I wrote down the license plate numbers of the parked vehicles before we drove away.

The fog thinned as we dropped lower in altitude. The first populated place we could stop was the grocery store at the turnoff to the Alyeska Ski Area. Lynn wouldn't get out. "I won't leave you but will be ready if you come running."

"We have to report this."

"I know, but I'm shaking so much I can't walk."

I walked up the wooden steps and entered the store, thinking that we had seen a lot of dead people in our work and that Lynn was overreacting. I waited while the young woman at the counter helped an older couple. When they left, I blurted out, "I need the police right away. There's a body along Crow Creek Pass Trail."

She screamed. "Oh, no! My sister didn't come home last night. We've been worried sick. Is it a man or a woman?"

"It's a young woman."

She jerked the phone off the hook and dialed, raving as she waited for someone to answer. "God damn her. If she wouldn't pick up with just any good-looking guy and shoot drugs, she wouldn't get herself in trouble. It's probably not her anyway. Misty's too damn mean to die."

She handed the phone to me.

"Alaska State Patrol."

"Hello. This is Dr. Kelly McKay. My friend and I just came off Crow Creek Pass. There is a body of a young woman beside the trail, partially clothed and bloody. I think it's a homicide, and there are hikers on the trail, including a child."

"Hang on, Doctor. I need some details, but I'll put out a call first."

I heard her make a radio call. "We have a body on Crow Creek Pass Trail, possible homicide. Others may be at risk. Please respond."

She returned to me. "Please spell your name. Tell me exactly where you are. A trooper has been dispatched. I'll contact Anchorage Borough and the coroner. Please stay where you are so you can direct them."

I gave her the details of what we had seen and about the other people on the trail and then hung up.

The store clerk dialed the phone. "Mom, come down here right away." Her voice trembled. "Somebody found a body along the trail. It might be Misty."

I heard a shriek and a click.

"I'm so sorry. I hope it's not your sister."

"So do I. My mother's an alcoholic. This will send her over the edge." The clerk made a couple more phone calls.

I bought two Cokes and went to the door. "I'm going outside. My friend is in the car. The police asked us to wait here."

Lynn opened the door when she saw me coming down the steps toward the car.

I got in, closed the door, and locked it. "The troopers are en route. We need to stay here and show them where the body is located."

Lynn shook her head. "I don't want to go back out there. This is a fine way to end your first real day of vacation in Alaska."

I said nothing for a few minutes. "The teenager at the cash register in there thinks it's her sister who didn't come home last night."

Lynn checked the door lock. "I'm scared. What if he was out there last night? Maybe having those guys stay at the cabin saved our lives."

"Yeah, but maybe they killed her."

"They were harmless college guys. Charming."

"So was Ted Bundy."

I thought for a moment. "You and the guys were snoring when I heard a piercing scream. It was far away." I added, "We don't know what time they left. I didn't hear them." The recollection sent a chill through my body. "I thought it was a marmot. Maybe it was her."

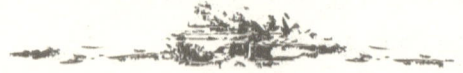

After about half an hour, two Alaska state trooper cars pulled in beside us. Lynn and I got out of the car to talk with them. After a short conversation, they decided one of us should stay with a trooper and talk with the store clerk. Lynn volunteered, leaving me to direct the investigators to the body.

I didn't mind. I had always been interested in forensics and had learned a lot working with Seattle Detective Cy Jones on cases in the Harbor ER. Somehow, this was worse, away from the protection of the hospital.

I got in with the trooper and rode to the trailhead parking lot. On the way, he said, "The coroner and Anchorage police are en route. They'll meet us in the parking lot and you can take us to the body."

I felt comfortable with the trooper; at least he had a gun. I wished I had mine with me. I should have carried it on the hike. We were far from town and had felt comfortable. The thought had not crossed my mind that anyone would follow us, nor that there was any danger except from wildlife.

Two cars remained. The van had disappeared. I gave the officer my note with the license numbers, including the missing vehicle. He called in an all-points-bulletin just as a black-windowed Suburban and an unmarked car arrived. A familiar figure emerged from the Suburban, the coroner who had come to the ER a few nights earlier.

The trooper asked me to describe the situation to the newcomers. Then he stayed behind to close the road and trail while the four of us walked toward the trailhead. The detectives walked ahead with caution.

I stayed a distance behind them with Dr. Ramsey, impressed with how easily the men trucked uphill once we reached the trail. I was half their age, out of breath, and unnerved.

Dr. Ramsey slowed his pace. "Are you okay?"

"As ER docs, my friend and I have seen a lot of trauma and blood. I'm surprised I feel so unnerved by this."

"You'd never expect to find a murder victim along this trail." His brow furrowed. "How's your friend doing?"

"Usually nothing fazes Lynn, but she's had a similar reaction to mine. We're both feeling uneasy this close to a murder way out here."

"Were you on a holiday hike?"

"Yeah. Stayed overnight at the summit. Taking a break and seeing the area. It's my first spring in Alaska." I explained we'd trained at the University of Washington, Harbor Medical Center in Seattle. "You came into the ER a few nights ago on a case."

"Right. That terrible shooting, but any place after Harbor is a piece of cake for you. How do you like being here, so far?" He hesitated. "I mean, before today."

"Good. We both like it."

"After Harbor, this ER is low key. Since you're new to Alaska, if you're interested in flying and getting to know the area better, I could take you for a flight sometime."

I told him about my new plane and my desire to fly a lot during the summer. "I'm still getting used to the Maule and would like to fly with you."

"Alaska is very unforgiving country."

I found it easier to talk at the slower pace he'd set. "I've been flying with the Civil Air Patrol, so I know what you mean. A lot of pilots get lost."

I looked up the trail and called to the detectives. "We're almost there. The body is just off the left side of the trail."

We had just reached the body when the little red-haired boy hopped down the trail in front of his grandpa and parents. I heard a giggle. The detectives shielded him from the body. We caught up and helped block the grisly scene.

The little boy's eyes widened when he saw all of us.

Dr. Ramsey walked down the trail a few feet and squatted down to talk. "Somebody got hurt along the trail. We came to see what happened." He motioned to the adults with him. "You can go on down to the parking lot. There's an officer down there who would like to ask you all some questions before you leave the area." The old man took his grandson's hand and walked ahead.

When the family was a distance away and out of view, the men started their evaluation of the scene. We walked closer to the body. Late morning sunlight penetrated the pine branches, casting shadows on the body. Wisps of fog hung in the trees, adding gloom to the scene.

Detective Rick Moore pulled a roll of yellow crime scene tape from his small backpack and cordoned off the trail, tying a yellow swath into the nearby woods.

Virgil Wescott, the second detective, pointed to marks at the edge of the rocky trail. "Looks like he dragged her off the trail here."

Detective Moore knelt near her head. "She looks familiar, but it's hard to tell for sure because of her injuries." He pulled a camera from his pack and, with the coroner, took close-up photos detailing the visible injuries, documenting body position and proximity to the trail. After scouring the area for evidence, the three men put on gloves and rolled the body onto an open body bag. The stiff limbs in rigor mortis resisted their efforts to zip the bag closed. One arm sprang toward Virgil, touching his pant leg. He jumped back.

Dr. Ramsey held the arm as the other two men closed the bag. "Which one of you is staying here to talk with other hikers coming down off the trail?"

"Unfortunately, it's me." Virgil shuddered, watching us leave. "We have to close the trail at both ends. Owners of the other cars may be coming from the cross-country route out of Eagle River. I've seen a lot of deaths, but this trail is spooking me. I'm glad the fog is thinning out."

Dr. Ramsey and Detective Moore lifted the bag by the loops at each end.

Detective Wescott lit a cigarette with a shaky hand as he watched us leave. He inhaled. "I hope I'm outta here before dark or that I get some company up here." His cigarette smoke blended into the fog.

I followed the men as they struggled with the awkward load down the rocky trail. At the Suburban, I opened the back door.

They hoisted the body in and Dr. Ramsey closed the door. "Rick, it's been a long day for Dr. McKay and her friend. Could they come into the station in the morning to give statements?"

Detective Moore handed me his card. "Could you show up about 9 a.m. at Homicide?"

Other police cars, some unmarked, and a number of men in street clothes milled around the parking lot. I wanted to leave and gladly got into the hearse with Dr. Ramsey when he invited me to ride back to the store with him.

Bouncing down the narrow road, the hair stood up on my arms when I heard the body thumping over the bumps.

A bad end to a great hike.

Dr. Ramsey looked over at me. His tousled dark hair magnified the contrast with his anemic skin, maybe pale from too many hours indoors looking at bodies. "Sorry this had to happen to you, Kelly, and to her."

"Thanks. I'll be okay. But I could sure use a drink." I meant water, but it came out wrong.

He laughed, "Something to calm your nerves, huh? Well, the Birdhouse is close by, but you and your friend should probably lock yourselves into a nice, warm, safe place till your nerves settle down. Send out for pizza."

"I meant a Coke, but anything sounds good right now. After a day like this, I'll be looking over my shoulder and acting paranoid if a stranger smiles at me."

"You'll get over this scare. Be sure to go on some more hikes."

He parked next to my car. I passed officers inside talking to the clerk and an older woman near the front of the store. When the officers saw Dr. Ramsey, they excused themselves to speak with him outside.

Lynn sat at a small table near a pop machine in the back. She got up and bought me a Coke. "You look like you need this. Can we leave now?"

We met an officer coming inside as we headed out. He talked to the mother and daughter. "I'd like one of you to look at the body and make an identification. If it's Misty, we need to know."

"Mom, I'll do it. Just come with me. Hold my hand and look away. I've never seen anyone dead before."

We walked to the door and waited for them to pass.

Dr. Ramsey opened the back.

The bell above the door rang as the door opened and rang again as it slammed shut, a death toll.

The older woman sobbed and gripped her daughter's hand as they approached Dr. Ramsey.

We waited outside the store.

Dr. Ramsey reached inside and opened the bag.

As if in a silent movie, the women bent forward and peered inside.

Mother's hand moved slowly to cover her face. Her body racked with sobs.

The daughter pulled her back. Their faces were streaked with tears as they stumbled back up the steps and past us. I opened the door for them.

The young woman said, "It's her. It's Misty. It's over, Mom. I worried about her all the time. Now we don't have to worry anymore. She's gone."

The older woman collapsed into a chair. The officer made arrangements with the younger woman to meet Dr. Ramsey at the hospital the following day to sign some forms. He suggested they close the store for the day or call someone to come in.

"I called an employee who is on his way. Would you take my mother home?" the clerk asked the officer. "We live together just up the road. I'll go home and stay with her as soon as I can leave."

Lynn and I told them we were very sorry about Misty and went out to talk to Dr. Ramsey. We found him securing the back door on his vehicle. I introduced Lynn.

"Pleased to meet you. I'll follow you ladies into Anchorage and make sure you get where you're going. I'll probably see you tomorrow at the police station or at the hospital. I'm the pathologist at the Regional Hospital and use the morgue there for forensic cases."

We got in and locked the doors. "Seems like a nice guy. He knows we're freaked out." Lynn peered into the back seat before fastening her seat belt.

"You checking to be sure we don't have a boogeyman in the back?"

Lynn punched my arm. "You might say that." I backed out and headed toward Anchorage. The Suburban followed within view. He waved and drove off when we parked at the apartment.

I still felt uneasy.

When we walked in, the sliding deck door was closed, but I still felt uneasy. I checked the lock. "Lynn, I know I locked this two days ago. It's unlocked."

"Maybe Dale was here and left it open. I'll ask him to keep us locked in. He's working. I need to call him."

I checked the windows to be sure they were locked before lying down for a nap. I had a fitful sleep with nightmares about flying in clouds, with the clouds swirling inside the cockpit and making it difficult to see. I was lost, searching desperately for a place to land. About midnight, I awakened and found Lynn cooking spaghetti. She couldn't sleep.

Every creak in the building startled us, but we finally went to bed.

The next morning, the helicopter lifting off from the hospital and flying over the apartment awakened me. Later, after showering and getting dressed, I awakened Lynn to get ready to go to the police department.

She startled so violently that I jumped back. "I can see we're both calm after a good night's sleep."

We stopped for espresso and a muffin en route to the police station.

Chapter 19 Homicide Investigation

I longed for a stout cup of Harbor Medical Center coffee with a shot of cream. Coffee that had caramelized after being left on the burner for about eight hours would be just about right. The double-shot latte I bought on the way to the homicide office wasn't strong enough.

We found our way in light morning traffic. If there were traffic jams in Anchorage, they had dissipated. Lynn gazed silently out the window.

I eased the car into a parking spot. "I'd rather be back in the trenches at Harbor Medical Center right now than dealing with bodies!"

"This is a sad interruption of our holiday fun. I feel sorry for the poor dead girl. Nobody deserves that."

"Since I was stabbed, this stuff really bothers me. It makes me shudder when that image of purple blurs of underwear, mottled skin, and fireweed keeps coming to mind. I hope I don't think of that death scene every time I see fireweed in bloom. It's such a beautiful flower."

"I saw her in my dreams last night. She was rocking and screaming on that damn sailboat being raped by my Uncle Bob." Lynn stopped. "He raped me when I was thirteen. You are the only one I've ever told. I hope he rots in hell."

I hugged her. "I'm so sorry."

"I was too ashamed to tell anyone. I felt so dirty. It has haunted me all these years. I wanted to confront him when I got older, but he's my mother's favorite little brother." We walked slowly toward the building. "I thought being this far away from home and this many years later, I'd forget about him. This stirred up bad memories. I wonder if she was raped, too."

"Now I understand why you didn't want to go back home. Why you are so negative about Boston. Just remember it's not your mother's fault, so don't take it out on her."

"I realize that, but she carries on about her wonderful brother who can do no wrong."

"There's the Suburban. Looks like Dr. Ramsey is already here."

We got out of the car. Lynn said, "I still don't believe this. What are we doing walking into a police station in Anchorage? You're supposed to be away from stress, having a great time in Alaska. Here we are making statements about a murder, and I'm whining about something that happened to me fifteen years ago."

We entered a large older building with noisy dark tile floors. "Brace up. You're strong as nails, and you know it. You grew up in that East Coast jungle of competition, and we survived Harbor Medical Center. Now we just need to remember all the details about one day to help them arrest the guy."

A young female in uniform at a desk gave us a quizzical look. "Could you direct us to Homicide?" She motioned us down a corridor to Rick Moore's office. *Homicide Division*, the door read uninvitingly.

The men sat talking to him when we walked in. Rick got up. "Good morning, ladies."

Dr. Ramsey poured us each more coffee. "I haven't done her post yet, but her primary visible injuries are ligature marks around her neck and a gash in her left thigh."

I suddenly felt faint and sat down.

Virgil Wescott walked in. "Does she faint at the sight of blood?"

Lynn stared at me. "What's with you Kelly? What's wrong?" She shook my arm.

"This sounds just like the girl I took care of in the ER a few nights ago. Identical injuries, including the jagged leg slash. You might want to talk to whoever investigated the assault. She was comatose on a ventilator last I knew."

"Unfortunately, Kelly, she died. I did her case yesterday. Her brain herniated from gross swelling, but the cause of death was asphyxia."

We wrote out our statements.

Detective Moore stood to see us to the door. "You are free to go. About those guys you met on the hike, an officer at the Eagle River parking area identified them when they drove in to pick up a car. We don't think they're involved. Thanks for your help.

"Dr. Ramsey, please call me to go flying with you sometime." I hesitated, not sure if he'd consider me brash. "How would you feel about me watching you do the autopsy? I've always been interested in forensics."

"I'd enjoy having you with me. No one admires my work." He made a fake frown. "Can you show up at my office at one thirty?"

Before we had gotten outside the building, Lynn lambasted me. "Kelly, you are nuts. Here you are afraid, having panic attacks in Seattle and nightmares here, and now you want to watch an autopsy on a homicide?" We reached the car and got in. "Count me out. I want to go home and lock the doors. One more day off, then back to work. Doubt if I'll leave the apartment till then."

Maybe Lynn had a point.

Chapter 20 The Flying Coroner

Antiseptic odors pierced my nostrils when we entered the autopsy suite. Bright overhead lights reflected from two gleaming stainless-steel dissection tables. Dr. Ramsey and I wore scrubs protected by fluid-impervious gowns. He handed me a pair of gloves. "Turns out Misty was a 17-year-old problem child. Alcohol, drugs, and prostitution."

"I got that impression from her sister. Their alcoholic mother adds to the sad family situation."

A gray-haired male assistant pulled out a refrigerated drawer. On the slab lay the familiar black bag I'd watched Dr. Ramsey and Detective Moore lug down the trail and slide into the black-windowed hearse. Today, the prominent protrusions from rigor mortis had relaxed. Instead of a bag with unusual lumps that could have been a bag of sports equipment, the silhouette looked like a body.

The assistant slid the bag to a gurney and wheeled the body to the dissection table, where he unzipped the bag. Seeing the exposed, lifeless body made me sad. The three of us positioned her partially clothed body in the center of the table.

Dr. Ramsey placed a block beneath her neck. "Dan, this is a homicide, so be extra careful with labeling."

"I getcha, Boss. I heard about this one on the morning news and knew we had our work cut out for us today. Who's your new friend?"

"Oh, sorry, I thought you knew everybody. Guess you'd only know Kelly if you were getting your healthcare in the ER. This is Kelly McKay. She is a new ER doc from Seattle."

"Kelly, meet Dan the Diener. He and I have worked together for years."

We exchanged hellos.

Dr. Ramsey said, "Kelly, call me Cornell. We're informal in my department. There are no patients to complain."

Dan smiled.

Ramsey dictated into a voice-actuated microphone attached to his collar. He explained to the transcriptionist that a guest physician was accompanying him and he'd be explaining things that should not to be included in the official report. "She's done transcription for me for years. She's so accurate, I hardly have to read her work. She'll know what to cut from my babbling and will leave in the appropriate details.

Cornell and I stood back while Dan took head and neck X-rays. We read the digital images as they appeared on a monitor. No fractures or deformities. No evidence of old healed injuries.

The thin body lay supine on the metal drain table. One hip and knee were slightly flexed, an arm was angulated, and a fist grasped green weeds. Her head was cocked to one side as if intently listening to Cornell as he dictated into the microphone. One non-seeing eye stared at the florescent light above the table. The rigor had softened enough for Cornell to force her limbs into alignment for the autopsy. He dictated the name, birth date, and case number.

"The body is that of a cachectic white teenage female. The decedent is wearing only a torn bra and purple bikini undergarments. No other clothing. Body weight, ninety-two pounds; height, sixty-five inches. Head hair is brown, extending one inch from the scalp, bleached blond beyond to earlobe length.

"Pupils fixed and dilated. Blue eyes, sclerae and conjunctivae show hemorrhagic changes consistent with petechiae over the face, with dense discoloration beneath each eye.

"Identification is by toe tag. The autopsy is not material to identification of the body.

"External findings include the following: A deep purple groove and torn skin around her neck consistent with ligature marks. Small nicks along the left neck near the shoulder are consistent with torture cuts. Scattered lacerations on fingers, palms, and dorsal forearms, consistent with defensive wounds.

"Three-centimeter tattoo of a red rose with a thorny green stem on anterior left chest. A metal ring in the left nipple. A stud in the navel, and a stud through her tongue.

"Left thigh laceration in the shape of the capital letter M."

Dan handed Cornell a ruler.

"The laceration measures eighteen centimeters in length, two centimeters in depth, hemorrhage into adjacent muscle tissue.

"Excoriations on the back and buttocks compatible with post-mortem injuries and insect activity.

"No visible signs of perineal trauma. Specimens are collected for forensic evaluations of secretions."

"Kelly, do you want to do the Y-incision?"

"Sure. Beneath the clavicles, then midline to the pubis?"

"Correct. I also want a midline neck incision to the chin to examine the ligature-injured area."

Cornell continued his dictation following my incision and our examinations. Inside, we found no gross pathology or injury to internal organs or structures.

"I performed this autopsy on the body of Misty June Arnold in the Pathology Lab at Regional Medical Center, Anchorage, Alaska, on May 31, 2015, at fourteen hundred hours. Her body was found near the trailhead of Crow Creek Pass by passersby. No information is available regarding the circumstances of her death. Based on multiple findings noted above, her cause of death is the result of asphyxia by garrote strangulation, a homicide. Laboratory studies are pending. End of dictation."

We stepped back and removed our gloves. Cornell took off his microphone. "Dan, will you take over and do the rest of the collections and see that Shelly gets the autopsy report done today?"

Dan agreed and continued placing labels on vials of blood and urine. He placed them into a container along with jars of formaldehyde with tissue samples Cornell dissected for documentation of the strangulation injuries in her neck.

"Kelly, I have an autopsy to do in Soldotna tomorrow. I'm flying down in my Super Cub. You're welcome to join me for the autopsy and get some flying in, too."

I hoped I could go. "I work at seven in the evening. Will you be back by then?"

"Figure we'll be gone two to three hours, max. You'll be back long before work, maybe by noon."

We agreed to meet at Peggy's Cafe for an early breakfast.

Cornell cautioned, "Bring a warm jacket with a hood. Flying in Alaska, you have to prepare for the worst. I've seen snow in July."

Chapter 21 Danger

Cigarette smoke hung in the air when I walked into the apartment after leaving Dr. Ramsey in his office. I wondered who'd been visiting Lynn. We didn't even have an ashtray in the house. "Hi, Lynn. Are you home?"

I pushed open the bathroom door. Pantyhose I'd left hanging over the shower curtain railing lay on the floor, the crotch shredded.

Cigarette ashes floated on the toilet water.

A shriek lodged in my throat. I ripped back the shower curtain.

Is someone in the apartment?

I spun around and looked in the bedrooms—both doors ajar, clothing strewn, linen ripped from the mattresses.

No one there.

My anxiety dropped, but fear for Lynn's life gripped my thoughts.

I rushed out of the apartment into my car and locked the doors. I called Lynn's cell. No answer. I drove to the hospital and stopped in the ambulance entrance. I left the car running and ran inside. "Have you seen Lynn?"

Nurses looked up from the desk. One said, "She's not due back till tomorrow morning. Dale's out on a flight, so she's not with him."

I went back outside and called Lynn again. Still no answer. I called Rick Moore at Homicide. "Rick, this is Kelly McKay," I said, my voice raspy.

"Hi, Dr. McKay, what can I do for you? Is something wrong?"

"I'm scared. Someone broke into our apartment, and I can't find Lynn."

"Maybe your roommate left it unlocked. Are you just jumpy after finding the murder victim?"

"No." Damn him for thinking I'm that squeamish. "Someone damaged the lock. Our apartment's trashed and her car is in the garage."

"Where are you?"

"Outside the Regional ER ambulance entrance."

"Stay there. I'll be there in a few minutes."

I dialed Lynn's cell and left another message.

When Detectives Moore and Wescott pulled up and got out, Virgil said, "We'll follow you to the apartment."

One of the men kicked open the apartment door, slamming it against the wall. They disappeared inside. Rick came back. "It's safe to enter, but the bedrooms are a mess. Underwear shredded, bras cut, drawers emptied. The bedding is scattered on the floor. It's definitely a pervert."

"I'm worried about Lynn. In Seattle, she attracted some strange characters."

"Try calling her again," Virgil suggested. "I hope it's not the guy who killed those other two girls. After seeing what that bastard does to women, until we get him, it concerns me having you or any woman out without a bodyguard."

Rick sat at the table and jotted down some notes. "What's Lynn's phone number, full name, and description?" He stood to leave. "My wife's visiting her mother in Oregon for a couple weeks. I may have her stay longer."

"Would Lynn have gone jogging or something?" Rick inquired.

"Maybe, but I thought I'd find her locked in and asleep."

As the detectives were leaving, a rattletrap International truck parked in a cloud of exhaust beside their unmarked car. Lynn got out carrying two bags of groceries in each hand.

The old truck drove off.

I ran out to meet her. The detectives followed. "We were about to go looking for you. I got back from the autopsy and found you gone. Where have you been?"

"I went for a walk about an hour ago and stopped to pick up a few things at the store. Why?"

Virgil pointed at the smoking truck. "Who drove you home?"

"I don't know his name. I met him at the hospital a few days ago, one of the new security guards. He offered to drive me home with all my groceries. I think I bought too much stuff. What's going on?"

"I'll carry some of your bags." Virgil offered. "Let's go in and talk about this situation."

Lynn looked aghast. "What situation?"

Virgil took two bags.

"Guys, I'm really sorry to cause trouble. I felt like taking a walk."

"Why didn't you answer your phone?"

"Dead battery. Why the fuss, Kelly?"

"Check out the apartment." Rick held open the door.

Lynn walked in and gasped. "Kelly who's been smoking in here? I hate cigarettes."

Rick's grim expression and gesture toward the bedrooms directed Lynn to look for herself. She left the groceries on the table and walked into her bedroom. She came back out and dropped into a kitchen chair, pale and shaken. "What a mess. Who did this?"

Rick asked, "Who else has a key?"

"My friend Dale Ayers. He's a pilot with the flight program and went out on a medical flight. He couldn't have been here and doesn't smoke."

Virgil announced, "You can't stay here. The lock is damaged."

I looked at the deck door. "The bar blocking this door is gone. Maybe he planned to return." A blurred image of the dead girl made me shudder. "Could the same guy be after us?"

"Maybe he planned to use the bar as a weapon. It won't be safe for you to stay here until you get a new lock installed—and you need a deadbolt. Is there someone you can stay with?"

"We can stay at Dale's place. Come on, Kelly, let's get some clothes together and leave with the detectives. Maybe he's still around watching."

Rick checked the damaged door. "Don't go anywhere alone and be sure to carry pepper spray. It could give you time to get away."

"Lynn, maybe the guy you got a ride with is okay, but many security guards are misfit cop wannabes. Don't accept rides from anyone," I begged. "Remember that security officer patient you took care of on the psych ward in Seattle?" I cringed. "He prowled around in uniform stalking women and ended up in prison for rape."

"This guy was in uniform, and I trusted him."

Chapter 22 Bush Flying

The morning paper's headline in the entrance to Peggy's Cafe stopped me: *Serial Killer*. I dropped in coins and bought the paper. I started reading as I waited to be seated. I'd finished the article and two cups of coffee by the time Cornell arrived. An older man followed him. I waved.

"Hi, Kelly. I brought Marty Phelps, a famous bush pilot, with me. I wanted you to meet him."

"Good morning, Doc." A short guy with a big smile, about seventy years old, sat across from me.

"I told Marty about you being a pilot and new to Alaska. He's the one who taught me bush piloting skills, and I wanted you to meet him and take a few lessons. It will save your life someday."

"Don't be scared of flying with me. I'm a hard-ass instructor who doesn't like his students killing themselves in airplanes." He grinned. "I've flown many an airplane in the bush—crashed a few, too. I'll teach you how to crash and survive. That's the true definition of a bush pilot, you know."

"Marty has no diplomacy. If you can stand him, he'll make it worth your time."

"I don't mince words Doc, but I like you already. If you want to give it a try, we're a team."

I felt a bit overwhelmed with the two guys talking about flying and not dying, one of them a coroner. Because my father had died in a plane crash, leaving me burned and broken, they didn't have to do a lot of talking to convince me to take a few more lessons. "Sounds good to me!"

"Heard you bought a Maule. That's a good plane. It's maneuverable and dependable."

The waitress showed up with menus. The men didn't look at them. I ordered French toast. Eggs, bacon, and hash browns didn't sound good. The men ordered "the usual," biscuits and gravy.

Marty poured cream and sugar in his coffee. "I'm retired, so my time is my own. I live in Talkeetna. Ma will feed the dogs, so I can come down and meet you any time, or you can fly up there. She let me outta town today to do some major grocery shopping. She's not much on flying, and it takes a couple hours to drive to Anchorage. I have to fly back down later in the week, if you want to fly with me then."

"I have three days off after working three nights beginning tonight. The timing is perfect."

Marty smiled. "I'll meet you here, Friday about noon."

Cornell and Marty cleaned their plates in record time. "I'm impressed. After years of medical training and eating on the run, there are very few who can beat me finishing a meal."

Marty said, "Stick with us, Kelly. We'll teach you a few other tricks, too." Cornell laughed at Marty's remark. I wasn't sure what he meant.

Cornell and I left Marty at the door. We both drove to Merrill Field and parked beside Cornell's Super Cub, which had large tundra tires, the kind the bush pilots use on off-field landings. We were airborne and southbound in minutes. "Summer mornings, there's often a line of planes waiting to leave. Today it's quiet. You can take the stick now if you'd like." Cornell let go. "Climb to fifty-five hundred feet. I like to fly a little high when I'm crossing Turnagain Arm. Once we're across, just follow the coastline around to the airport. It's a short flight."

I took the stick and craned around his neck to see the airspeed indicator and the altimeter, not the easiest procedure when flying a Cub from the back seat. Gray clouds hung low over the Chugach Range east of town. The visibility improved southward. We crossed the saltwater arm, and a white snow cone rose in the distance, much like Mount Rainier near Seattle. I asked Cornell its name.

"Mount St. Augustine. It's volcanic like most of the peaks around here. Erupted in the early seventies and dumped a load of ash on Anchorage. The sky turned black in midafternoon."

The tone of the engine decreased. "We're still pretty high, so I cut the power. I'll take over and let you know what I'm doing so you can anticipate what's happening. I'm adding carburetor heat and we'll slip in at an angle to lose altitude faster."

Cornell adjusted a few knobs, and the engine noise decreased further. "Marty taught me well. He'll intentionally chew on your ego now and then. Sounds like a grizzly, but he's a teddy bear and damn serious about precise flying at maximum performance. Take what he says seriously. It will keep you alive."

Those words again.

We flew downwind, turned the base leg, and then made the final approach. Cornell landed very short, soft, no bounce, and rolled forward to turn off at the first taxiway.

"That was a perfect landing."

Cornell laughed. "I wanted you to see how little runway this thing really needs."

"My first ride in a Super Cub was on skis. It was not as maneuverable as this."

"That's what I like about this one. It's slower with the big tires, so you can't get where you're going very fast, but it will get you in and out of some very tight spots. My wife doesn't like sitting tandem, says she only has a good view of the back of my head. She'd like us to buy a side by side."

"I agree with her. I like sitting beside someone rather than tandem. Each plane has its drawbacks."

"If you're the pilot, it doesn't matter. The Super Cub is versatile. Probably why Marty uses one to drop supplies to climbers on Denali. He makes many flights some days just ferrying things and people. It's his part-time summer job."

A hearse parked beside the fuel shack. A very tall man got out. He waved a slender arm to Cornell as we taxied in.

A young man came out of the fuel office. "How long are you staying, Doc?"

"About three hours. Can I tie it down right here?"

"This is fine. If you're in a hurry, I'll tie it for you."

"I'll get it. Thanks anyway. I have enough fuel this time so won't need any."

Cornell turned to me and spoke quietly. "One thing I've learned is to always tie down my own airplane and always be present when it's refueled. Two friends died because they trusted someone who screwed up. One of them got the wrong fuel. His engine quit and he crashed into the water. Left a wife and two kids."

The tall man walked up.

"Hi, Stretch. Want you to meet Dr. McKay. Kelly works ER at Regional, trained in Seattle."

"Hello, Dr. McKay, name's Rudy Thomas, mortician and director of the little funeral home here. Today I'm chauffeur, too. My hearse is your taxi. How was your flight?"

"Beautiful. Cornell showed off his skills to a novice pilot."

"He's like that. Always showing off." Stretch changed the tone of his voice, "Cornell, I just have the one body for you. It's a sad case. The toddler drowned when he fell in the freezing cold Kenai River without a life jacket. I get so damn mad when parents don't make their kids wear life jackets and seat belts. It just kills me to see the anguish they have to live with forever."

Rudy drove us to the funeral home in his luxurious old hearse. It reminded me of riding in the black limousine for my grandmother's funeral, which was an unpleasant thought because it reminded me that I was in a burn unit when my father was buried. I fingered the scars on my neck and face, reminders of bad times but also of the second chance I had to live on and fly safely. Moments of gloom on an otherwise special day.

On the way to the simple funeral home in the small town, Cornell explained, "In the rural areas of Alaska, it's common to do autopsies in funeral homes. The practice saves transporting bodies long distances at great expense. I carry a traveling kit with supplies, camera, jars with preservatives for specimens to analyze, and all the paperwork. If the death is suspicious, we transport the body to my lab in Anchorage."

The autopsy took less than an hour. The external exam showed post-mortem skin discoloration, but instead of bluish-gray coloration, the child's skin looked splotchy and pink. The color was strange. The child appeared to be asleep, not dead. "Cornell, why is the skin so pink?"

"Cherry-pink livor is seen in bodies recovered from water and wearing clothing. You'll see it on bodies lying on moist covered trays, too. Humidity prevents escape of oxygen and allows for an excess of red oxyhemoglobin to remain in the skin."

"I thought we just saw that with carbon monoxide poisoning."

No, you'll see a similar pink color if someone dies of cyanide and other poisons." He moved the small limbs. "The stiffness of rigor mortis is still present. Hypothermia and cold temperatures slow chemical reactions and slow the rigor process. If we had ninety-degree temperatures outside, the rigor mortis would disappear within hours."

Silt in the mouth and stomach, with airways clear, confirmed no aspiration of river water. "Often when a child hits cold water, laryngeal spasm occurs and closes the airway, called the diving reflex. No aspiration of water occurs. The child dies without oxygen. It is a hypoxic death and considered a drowning even though there is no water in the lungs."

A careful exam for external signs of injury revealed nothing. The little boy had asphyxiated in the milky waters of the Kenai River. I felt weak looking at the sad loss of life.

I could never work as a pathologist.

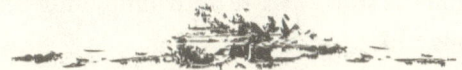

The touchdown at Merrill Field after a straight-in approach to runway 03 from the south was smooth. Cornell taxied to the Super Cub's tie-down, turned on a dime, and cut the engine. We got out and pushed the plane back into its parking site. Cornell tied each knot and locked the door. I watched.

"Locking the doors slows thieves down a little. I've never had a problem, but I know pilots who have lost radios. There is no security at Merrill Field. It's wide open." He added, "That's why a careful preflight check is important. You never know what goof has been playing around the plane since your last flight."

He added as we walked to our cars, "I always look for bird nests, too. Birds think of planes as condos. I fly mine enough that no feathered friends have time to take up residence."

"You fly like a professional."

"You'll be just as good when Marty gets done with you."

"I made it through organic chemistry and a thoracic surgery rotation with a madman, so I think I can take whatever Marty has to give me."

"You won't be sorry."

"Thanks for the interesting day. I better head home and take a nap before work. I hope the landlord got the locks changed so I can sleep at home."

"Why are you changing the locks, Kelly?"

I told him the story. "We're both jumpy after finding that body and now this break-in."

"That story worries me. Who could have been in your apartment?"

"I don't know. I thought at first it might be a former boyfriend from Seattle, a surgeon turned drug addict who showed up on my doorstep a few days ago. I came to Alaska to get away. He'd never trash the apartment like we found it."

"It doesn't sound good. I think I should follow you home."

"If you have time, I'd appreciate it. You had me so distracted with the flight and all, I forgot to tell you."

Outside the apartment, everything looked okay. We went to the landlord's apartment on the second floor. I rang his doorbell. Heavy footsteps approached, and the door opened a crack. "Oh, hello, Dr. McKay." He opened the door wide. "The lock man just left. He changed the door handle assembly that was jammed and put in a deadbolt like Dr. Cabot ordered. I cut off an old broom handle to block the deck door. Put it there myself." He handed me the keys. "The lock man will bill you for his work and the new locks."

Cornell and I went back downstairs. I tried the new keys. He said, "Carry pepper spray in your hand when you're outside. Don't go anywhere alone at night."

I felt exhausted and empty inside. After eating a box of macaroni and cheese, I slept a few hours and awakened to the alarm at 6 p.m., not ready to face the ER for twelve hours.

Chapter 23 New Flight Instructor

Lynn completed her patient report just as Dale walked into the ER and put his arm around her. "Is my pretty girl ready to go?"

"I'm ready." Lynn turned to me. "I've been uneasy all day thinking about the sicko who ransacked our apartment. I didn't want to be alone, so Dale is staying with me."

"I'm bringing Lynn back to work in the morning to relieve you, Kelly. Would you like a ride home? I'll make sure you're locked in for your beauty sleep."

"Sounds good. The incident freaked me out." Dale could be so nice.

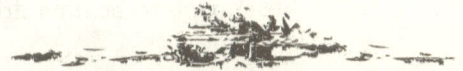

Work remained calm for the next few days, and my worries about being alone or followed decreased. Instead, my thoughts returned to getting more experience flying with Marty. Vic commented on my cheery attitude. I rushed around during my twelve-hour shifts, happily getting my charting and patient care finalized so I could leave on time. I told him my plans.

"Good. A few years ago, one of our doctors disappeared while flying in the winter without survival gear. After days of looking for him, the Civil Air Patrol called off the search. He's never been found."

Vic's words sent a jolt through me, instilling a stronger desire to fly safely. Later, over lunch at Peggy's, Marty described his lesson plan. "I want you comfortable in your own plane. Fly me around. Do a few touch-and-gos at Merrill, then land at Birchwood."

Knowing this gnarly expert would watch my every move made me tense.

"You know how to fly. I want see what I can do to improve your skills."

At Merrill Field, Marty climbed into the right seat. "Fly as if you were alone." He sat there with his hands folded in his lap, his feet light on the rudder pedals, watching and feeling every move I made as I talked to the tower and took off. He looked comfortable enough to be on a drive in the country.

After the approach and landing at Birchwood, Marty said, "You're an attentive, smooth pilot and have demonstrated to me you are a safe flier. Have you done any grass or dirt strip landings?"

"A few at a field at the Arlington airport north of Seattle."

"You know how it feels, then. Easy in a taildragger."

Easy for him to say.

"Could you come stay with me and Ma for a couple days? I'd take you out to do some off-field landings near Talkeetna."

"I want to get started doing the tough stuff right away. I could come up tomorrow."

"It's not tough. It's a matter of attitude. You already have the skill and brains. I'll show you the icefields and we'll land on some sandbars."

"Sounds scary. How do I find you when I get to Talkeetna?"

"We have two airports in town. I live on the south end of Talkeetna Village sod strip near downtown. Overfly once. I'll hear you on the radio and will come out to meet you. Park beside my Super Cub."

After Marty left, I flew for two more hours, refueled, and went shopping to stock the plane with survival gear for the 85-mile flight the following morning. Recent distractions had kept me from buying groceries, washing clothes, and reading mail. Paying the eighty-five-dollar bill for the locksmith smarted, but everything in Alaska cost more.

A letter from sister Kris carried good news. Her marriage was off. She had dumped the unreliable bastard. I had never met the guy, but I didn't like him. I'd hoped she'd be better at choosing men than I. Dumping him was a start.

I threw a load of junk mail in the garbage on top of numerous empty beer cans.

Shit. Dale was drinking again.

Chapter 24 Alaskan Bush Flying

The restricted airspace of Elmendorf Air Force Base blocked a direct route to Talkeetna, but once clear of the area, I flew IFR northward along the Parks Highway. A joke among pilots is that IFR means *I follow roads*. IFR really stands for instrument flight rules, which means flying in clouds under radar control without ground visibility. But for many private pilots, using roads as landmarks makes navigation easy, and, if engine problems occur, a road provides a very long landing strip.

I didn't need a GPS to tell me the route but set it up for practice. My new backpack, filled with organized survival gear, sat within reach on the seat behind me. It would do me no good to have freeze-dried food, protein bars, Snickers, peanut butter, and Fig Newtons that could keep me going for days if they were out of reach. Placing the backpack in the storage area would make it out of reach for emergency access after a crash. I'd tucked in a small hatchet and a package of fishing supplies for good measure. My down jacket, with a plastic shelter and knife in one pocket and a lighter in the other, lay on top of the pack.

I slid my .32 Walther PPK handgun into the pocket in the seat back on the passenger side and fastened my seat belt.

I touched down on the sod strip about an hour after leaving Anchorage.

Marty, flanked by two beautiful, gangly gray dogs, walked out to meet me at the tie-down area. The dogs' intelligent faces bore dark masks like huskies. They circled him happily, jumping and pawing each other until they neared me. Then, on hand command, each one stayed at his side on heel.

"Hi, Kelly. We'll be flying my plane, so let's tie this down even though there is no wind. We'll be taking off right after you meet Martha. First, meet Tal, my wolf mix named for the Talachulitna River, one of my favorite places. The smaller one is Sue, for Little Mount Susitna, another favorite place." He released them. "They're from the same litter, half husky, half wild. It's that wild side I've tried hard to control. Without full control, they can be dangerous animals."

The wary animals sniffed and circled me. Strange golden eyes locked on mine. I tensed, but with Marty close by, they didn't frighten me. I held out a hand for them to sniff.

Marty put his arm around me. "Tal, Sue, this is Kelly. She's one of the pack. Guard! Guard!"

They wagged and moved closer, following us into the house.

"I fly a lot and leave Martha alone. They'd kill anyone who tried to hurt her."

We entered the small home into an open living room with dark pine walls where a potbelly stove sat in one corner. Pictures of Alaska adorned the walls. In the adjacent kitchen area, Martha, a small woman with gray hair in a ponytail, wearing a red sweatshirt and jeans, waved us in. "Come on in and have a cup of coffee before you take off. I'm fixing moose stew for lunch."

Marty introduced us. He lifted the cover on a stew pot for me to see the bubbling broth filled with dark meat and veggies. It smelled delicious.

"Moose is a staple around here. I harvest one every year. We eat it almost every day and give a bunch away." We sat at the table and Martha joined us. "What time do you want us back?"

"How about noon? That'll give the vegetables time to cook." She motioned toward a hallway off the living room. "Your bed is ready, but I need to clean up this place. Our overnight company just left."

"Now, Ma, don't be fretting about the house. It looks fine. We'll be flying along the Susitna River toward Curry. You'll know where to look if we're late for lunch." She hugged him as we went out the door. Tal and Sue remained with Martha.

I smiled. They reminded me of Lucille and Ed Jensen, dogs and all.

Marty put me in the back of his Super Cub and then climbed in. "Keep your hand on the stick and your feet on the rudder pedals to give you a feel for what I'm doing."

It felt cramped. I could see nothing but the back of his head when looking forward, like when I flew with Cornell and Hugh up in McGrath.

The visibility out the side windows was fine for sightseeing but not for piloting.

We flew about five hundred feet above the water, snaking northward too low to have any time to choose a place to land if the engine quit. Marty reduced power and circled lower.

He said he was setting up for a landing along the water. He dipped a wing. "Our landing site is that level sandy spot, the sandbar, along the river.

We came in low and slow. He talked me through his technique and emphasized the importance of knowing the landing area. "If you get mired down, there is no one out here to help. You're on your own." I recalled his instructions to Martha. "Always tell someone where you are going so if you don't return, eventually someone will come looking, just in case you screw up and can't take off or crash somewhere."

Marty demonstrated a short-field takeoff. After a few bumps, he horsed the plane into the air long before I thought it was ready to fly. He chose a couple more sites and landed, each time explaining why he had chosen the particular spot. The third was the widest and the smoothest. "Let's get out and walk around a little so you can see this backcountry up close." He was out and looking into the rushing water before I could climb out of the back.

It was silent except for the sound of water rippling over rocks and a jay announcing our arrival.

Peace. Here in remote Alaska, far from city noises and ER turmoil, I found peace.

Marty's voice broke the solitude.

"The winter melt and glacier runoff turns the river milky like you see now. In the fall, the water is lower, and the sandbars are wider, better for landing."

I squatted near the river and dipped my fingers in. "Oh, that's cold."

"Not swimming temperature, but I've bathed in it hundreds of times. Get pretty rank in hunting camp if you don't wash up." He fanned an armpit. "This is great moose hunting territory. If you come up during hunting season, we could get you a moose."

I wondered what I'd do with a whole moose. Maybe he and Martha would give me a package of burger instead. I couldn't kill such an amazing animal.

"We'd fly in and camp overnight. Can't fly and shoot on the same day or Fish and Game gets your airplane, gear, everything. I'd never do that anyway. There is no sport in it." Marty checked his watch. "We need to start home for lunch and a little nap before we head to Denali." Marty climbed into the back seat. "Now it's your turn to show me how it's done. Don't forget what I said about habitual airspeed control."

My feet trembled on the rudder pedals. "I'm not sure I'm ready for this. Can you land it from the back seat?"

"I can, but I won't need to. In fact, I want you to take off, climb out over the river till you are at five hundred feet, then line up and fly a pattern just like you would when landing at Merrill Field, only this time land right here on Kelly's sandbar."

My heart pounded, and my fingers went numb gripping the stick. We did four round trips. Landing, back-taxiing in the hard sand, and then another takeoff.

"See, you're getting the hang of it." Marty's calming voice added to the confidence I'd gained in just one morning.

Exhaustion compounded by a full stomach left me sleepy after lunch. I helped Martha with the dishes.

"I hope you aren't offended. We have this little habit of taking an afternoon nap. We don't mean to desert a houseguest, but Marty and I are up all hours. We never get to bed before midnight."

"I'm tired, too. Marty really gave me a workout. Wake me when you get up."

"There's a wool afghan on the couch. Curl up on the soft couch right by the stove and you'll be asleep in no time."

I sat on the couch, removed my boots, and then stretched out beneath the blanket.

"Tal, here boy," Martha called the big dog and pointed to the floor beside me. "Take care of Kelly. Stay."

I rested my hand on his furry back.

Tal turned and looked at me with intelligent eyes. Weird eyes. Wild eyes. His tail gave two thumps. When I quit petting him, he put his head down.

After the nap, Marty and I took my plane on a scenic flight over Ruth Glacier and overflew an area of relatively smooth snowfields, the drop-off place for Denali climbers. Winds rocked the wings. In the four-place Maule, Marty sat beside me. He pointed out the climbing route. "Gusts are too strong to risk landing any plane here today." Marty directed me to gain altitude. "We have to stay higher because of vicious up- and downdrafts near the mountains."

Marty told stories of rescues and hunting experiences as he directed me to various locations. He had me totally distracted when, without warning, he reached over and pulled off the power. "Your engine just quit. Where're you going to land?"

I didn't expect this test of emergency procedure, but after flying with my dad and many instructors, my response was automatic. I pointed to a sandbar I'd already identified as a possible landing site.

"Good choice. The rough brush on the tundra is never a good choice."

We went over forced landings time and time again. Marty's voice drummed, "Kelly, always fly the airplane. No matter what else is going on, fly the airplane." This was the same message my had father imprinted on my brain when I was a teenage pilot.

Marty's voice again: "A door blows open, a radio quits, and some pilots just quit thinking—and quit flying. It kills 'em. You're in charge. Nobody's going to do it if you don't. Remember that."

Marty talked constantly. I think to distract me from what I was doing. He'd ramble on and on, and then *wham*, he'd do something else to surprise me. I became wary, on guard, and was tempted to keep my hand on the throttle so he couldn't pull it out and cut power again. The two days of his teaching were invigorating but exhausting. The final day, he had turned to peer out his window when he abruptly turned back and blew cigar smoke in my face. "Fire in the cockpit."

Dang! My heartbeat stumbled and I thought I'd pee my pants. My hands shook. I shut down electronics, radios, checked the fuel, pulled off the power, and looked for a place to land. It was more realistic than I ever wanted to experience. It took an instant to run through the emergency plan, pretending I didn't know Marty was cause of the problem.

Marty was dead serious.

"Good. You didn't lose your cool." He wrinkled his nose and grinned. "You're a damn good pilot. You'll be the best lady pilot in Alaska when I get done with you and better than most men. When are you coming back for more?"

"In five days, after another four days of work."

"Call when you are coming. I'll have some real fun planned for the next time."

On my flight to Anchorage, I practiced saying emergency procedures aloud like I'd learned so long ago with Dad and now from Marty. Both voices replayed, "Watch that approach airspeed. Sixty-five. Not sixty-six. Sixty-five, damn it, sixty-five. It will save your life."

Chapter 25 Seeing Forever

Lynn looked up from stirring spaghetti sauce. Her perturbed expression and words surprised me. "What are you doing back so soon? I didn't expect you until tomorrow."

"I have to work in the morning." Lynn checked my work schedule taped to the refrigerator. "I misread it. I asked Dale to stay with me tonight after getting one of those damn phone calls."

The fear in her eyes spiked my concern. "Did you recognize the voice?"

Lynn shook her head. "A disguised male voice asked for a key to the apartment, saying he'd show me a good time." She put three plates on the table. "I slammed the receiver down, but not before I heard him laugh. I wonder if he knew you were gone. He specifically called you the last time."

"That means he knows both of us."

The toilet flushed, and Dale appeared in the doorway. Dale did a fake punch at the air. "I'd take care of him if he showed up here. He'd be a sorry son of a bitch."

His disheveled hair and slurred words told me why Lynn didn't want me home.

"Come on and eat. It's ready." Lynn served the food. "I think we should tell those detectives."

"I'll call them tomorrow." I checked the doors to be sure they were locked before sitting down. "Somebody is watching us."

Dale stumbled to the table. He disgusted me, but I'd sleep better with a surly guy in the house, drunk or not. "Two good-looking women attract attention, sometimes the wrong kind. Any problems with the new plane?"

"No problems." I told him about the lessons with Marty Phelps, flying his Super Cub and landing on sandbars along the Susitna River. "I like your instructor friend Tab, too. I figure the more people I fly with, the better."

"I agree. Just don't go landing on sandbars by yourself."

Lynn poured herself a glass of red wine and offered me some. "So, when will you take me flying again, Kelly?"

Dale opened a can of beer.

"Any time we're both off work. I've been looking at maps and talking to people about some real Alaskan spots with airstrips." I gladly accepted the wine. Its calming effects would put me to sleep and reduce my adrenaline level after the tense flying lessons and anxiety over yet another disturbing phone call. "Marty mentioned Hot Dam Hot Springs near the Arctic Circle."

"I've heard of it," Dale said. "An eight-hour drive from Fairbanks by dirt road, a nice gravel runway. If you want to experience the real Alaska, you found the right place. Very isolated." Dale mentioned a few more places Lynn and I might like to visit.

Our discussions at the table remained light. I didn't mention Dale's drinking. Lynn's stiff body language made me wonder if I'd walked in on an unfinished argument, now stilted by my presence. I excused myself and went to bed, where loud voices interrupted my sleep.

The following day began a stretch of shifts that kept me running. With longer hours of daylight and more tourists pouring into town in buses, each shift a few vacationers arrived with various ailments and forgotten medications.

Escaping to Talkeetna on my days off provided distraction and relief from work.

I had to give Marty credit for creativity. After the last flight before returning to Anchorage, he said, "Well, Kelly, I have enjoyed flying with you so much, I really don't want it to end. I have a meeting in Anchorage on Monday. Do you want to fly again with me then?"

We made arrangements to meet at my plane on Monday after lunch.

After we were airborne on Monday afternoon, Marty said, "Cross the inlet. I want to show you something."

"Where are we going?"

"I'll let you know when we're closer. We're going to see if a Maule can do what it's supposed to. I read the book. We'll be testing its limits." He cinched his belt tighter. "I told Cornell our destination. Remind me to call him when we get back, otherwise he said he'd come looking for us."

What did the two of them have planned?

"Keep climbing. I want you to go up to four thousand feet. Fly along the edge of Cook Inlet a ways, then go north around Mount Susitna."

I followed his instructions. When we approached the mountain, Marty announced, "Kelly, we're landing at Little Mount Susitna International." He laughed.

"Dale and I flew over it. I don't remember seeing an airstrip."

"It's not busy enough to waste the ink on a map. We'll come in from the north."

"Are you going to land this thing on a mountaintop?"

"Nope. You are. Good experience. Like always, I want you to overfly the landing strip first and examine it carefully. Try to tell which way the wind is from. For this landing, no matter what the wind, there's only one way to land, north to south." I paid attention to the flying but cast a questioning glance his way.

"You'll see why. It's on an incline. You land downhill. Then, you back taxi to the top to take off downhill."

We rounded Susitna. I looked for a runway, but I still didn't see one. "Where is it? Where's the runway?" I dipped a wing and scanned the ground near the top of the gently sloping mountain.

"We aren't close enough. Keep looking."

I looked down and shook my head. "Where is it?"

"Kelly, you have to hallucinate a little to see this one."

I circled and flew back over Little Sue. "Now, dip your left wing and look straight down. You'll see a white Clorox bottle. That marks the threshold. Be ready to touch down just to the right of the bottle."

"Are you kidding?"

"Nope. It's one of the best runways around here."

"For a mountaintop, I suppose you're right." I thought he was joking.

"For these real short ones, you want to do a full-stall landing. Airspeed control is essential. It's real short, so you must brake immediately on touchdown. Just do it firmly, not hard or jerky. You could nose over and damage the prop."

Shit. Marty is serious. Or is he? Maybe this is a test to see if my judgment is sound.

His calm voice directed me, "Get your pattern set up just like you would at a big airport except almost land about twenty yards short of the bottle, adding enough power to fly level. Chop the power when you get there."

I tried to do exactly as he said, knowing I could add power to gain altitude and abort at any time.

I touched down just a little before the white plastic jug. I braked with shaky legs. Soon the tires were bumping over the hummocks.

We came to a complete stop and I took a deep breath. I gripped my thighs to stop my hands from shaking.

With a very large grin on his face, Marty exclaimed, "Congratulations! You just passed your final exam. Now, taxi back to the top and let's get out to look at the view."

I stood on the top of the rounded mountain, rotating slowly three hundred and sixty degrees. The view went on forever.

My eyes followed Cook Inlet out to sea. Water met sky and became one.

Far below and across the inlet, tiny Anchorage reflected bright flashes of sun from high-rise buildings. The Chugach wall was to the east. Denali and Foraker rose like ice cream cones to the north. The Alaska Range rimmed the westward view. I had tears in my eyes when I finished the circle. "Is this heaven? Marty, I think we're in heaven." I gave him a bear-hug. "I can't thank you enough."

I sat on a rocky slope scanning the unobstructed view and cried. When I could speak, I hugged and thanked him again. "This is the best experience of my life."

He sat beside me. "Helluva pilot. You're one helluva pilot." He pointed to Denali. We still have to land you at the supply camp at the base of Denali. It will round out your skills." He stood. "Now, after we walk over the area where you will take off, about a hundred feet, tell me what your plan is to get me back to town."

We walked over the uneven terrain counting our steps, measuring the distance. I reviewed short-field takeoff technique.

"This is really short," he said. "It's a Super Cub strip. Minimum takeoff roll for the Maule is 150 feet, but we have half fuel. You and I are both on the light side, so I know it will be okay, but realize, we're cuttin' it close."

We got in and fastened our shoulder straps and seat belts tight. I taxied uphill on the rough ground, beyond the Clorox bottle as far back as I could go, and then pointed the nose downhill.

Marty talked me through it. "Give it a notch of flaps. Keep your toes on the brakes until you get full power. While holding the brakes push the throttle full forward."

The engine came to life. The plane shuddered. I locked the brakes.

Marty spoke calmly, "Hold. Hold. Hold. Okay!" He raised his voice, "Now, off the brakes! Let her roll. Forward pressure. Get the tail up. Watch your speed but look outside. Fifty-five. Okay, now gently pull back. I think she's getting ready to fly."

The plane barely lifted. "Keep her level. Nose down a hair. Pick up some airspeed. Fifty-six. Fifty-eight. Sixty. Sixty-five. Now she's climbing."

I looked down. The ground dropped away rapidly as we eased off the summit. "I can't believe we did this, Marty."

"You did it. I'm proud of you. You are a safe pilot, and now you have even more skill."

I relaxed. Climbed higher.

"Don't be foolish. Pay attention and always remember . . . fly the airplane. Let's go home."

Chapter 26 Overdue

A busy night shift ended and I walked home scanning for the unknown annoying man. I heard the phone ringing as I unlocked the apartment door. I rushed to the wall phone in the kitchen, leaving the door ajar. The voice said, "Kelly, is that you?"

"Yes. Is that you, Marty?" I hoped he wanted to fly again.

A muffled male voice, "Dr. McKay, why are you out of breath? You must be tired. You work too hard. When I think of you, Kelly, you make me hard."

"Who are you? Stop calling, damn you, or I'll report you to the police." I slammed the receiver down, slammed the door closed, and locked it.

Not safe in my own house.

The phone rang.

The answering machine picked up. "Kelly. Oh, Kelly, I know you're there. I like it when you're mad."

Who the hell would do this? There were so many mentally unstable people I'd met in the ER. It could be Birdman, but it didn't sound like him. I called the homicide office and talked with Detective Moore. He sounded concerned and provided guidance, same old stuff.

In the late afternoon, I called Dale. I thought he was probably up by then, like I was. He wasn't. I let the phone ring and ring. No answer. I checked the flight schedule Lynn had taped to our refrigerator door. Dale was on night call. To decrease lift-off delays, all helicopter pilots on first call had to remain at the hospital.

Lynn was not going to be happy about our getting another phone call.

I walked to the hospital, arriving right at change of shift, and found Dale with Lynn at the desk. I told him my great news. "Dale, I am so pumped. Marty gave me my so-called final exam. It's the most exciting thing I've ever done."

"What did he make you do?"

"I landed the Maule on Little Susitna."

"You're out of your mind and he's out of his friggin' mind to have you do it. Nothing bigger than a Super Cub on tundra tires should land there! You'll kill yourself doing foolish stuff like that, Kelly."

"It's the shortest airstrip I've ever seen, but the risk was worth it." I took a breath, flung out my arms, and spun 360 degrees. "The view was indescribable. Someday, I'd like to camp on top."

Lynn jumped up and down. "You, little old you, actually landed your plane up there?"

I nodded, grinning ear to ear.

Dale rounded his shoulders. "Now you've got it in your blood. More power to ya. Keep up the good work, just be careful."

"Thanks for helping me get the Maule. It was a good choice."

Dale shook his head. "Oh, my God. What have I done? Now the little lady is a bush pilot."

"I wouldn't go that far. To qualify as a bush pilot, according to Marty, you have to crash and live to talk about it. I'm happy without that title."

Dale started for the door and then turned back. "I see your point. I've never heard it put quite that way. I'm on helicopter call, so I'll be out there in my little room sleeping if you don't disturb me with flight call." He frowned. "I also have a shitload of paperwork to get done for the flight program. We have some inspections coming up."

"Rob Lewis was on last night. If he's on tonight, you won't get any sleep. He always has flights. I don't know how he arranges it. Luck, I guess."

He came back and kissed Lynn on the top of the head as she sat at the desk. "There's a storm offshore heading this way. Heavy rain, winds, and a low ceiling by morning. Doubt if we'll be flying. Bye. I'm going to bed."

After Dale left, I said, "We got another phone call."

Lynn stared at me. "You mean an obscene one?"

"Not really obscene, but yes. Another call from that guy, whoever he is." Lynn looked worried but got up to leave.

I said, "If he calls again tonight, call me. When I notified Rick Moore about getting more calls, he suggested changing our phone number."

"I don't want him to think we're a couple of ninnies who can't take care of ourselves. I'll call you when I get home, so you aren't fretting about me all night."

Lynn was still in ER when a radio call came in for a critical injury from a car accident. She helped me stabilize the man and get him to the operating room. Another accident victim from a motorcycle vs. a car arrived. We both followed ambulance personnel and ER nurses into the next trauma room. During the care of a critical trauma patient, it was nice to have extra help. Within seconds of our arrival, the young man said, "Oh, God, I'm dying."

And—he did.

We worked on him for an hour but never got him back. Lynn removed her gloves and protective gown. "I'll let you do the paperwork since I have to be back in the morning."

I worried about her going home alone. She called a few minutes later to inform me she'd made it.

Adding to the ER chaos, I answered a call on the flight phone. "The manager at Eureka Lodge about 90 miles east of here has a guest with chest pain."

Rob made calls to inform Dale and check the weather. "Dale says it's a go. The storm is approaching from the west, but we'll be back before it gets here."

The helicopter lifted off a few minutes later with Rob, a flight EMT, and Dale. Rob explained before they left, "Eureka Lodge is northeast of here past Gunsight Mountain, through Chickaloon and Tahneta Passes. We've been there a few times. Some rugged territory without good radio contact. We just follow the highway. I'll update you when we get there. Be back in a couple hours."

After they left, we were short two of our staff. It seemed busier than ever. I lost track of time. At 2 a.m., I realized they hadn't called. I asked the secretary. "What time did they leave?"

"It's been about two hours."

"We should have heard from them. Call Eureka Lodge and see when they left." She found the number, dialed, and handed the phone to me. After about the tenth ring, a voice answered irritably. I said, "Hello, this is Dr. McKay in Regional Medical Center ER. What time did the helicopter leave?"

"Leave? They haven't arrived." The voice was still irritated. "This guy is really sick, hardly conscious. I thought they'd be here an hour ago."

"If they haven't arrived, there must be a problem. They're overdue."

"You're damned right they're overdue. We need some help. He's got heart trouble. Said he was having another heart attack. When are they going to get here?"

I tried to remain calm and also calm him.

My mind raced. "Sir, you don't understand. If the helicopter hasn't arrived and we haven't heard from them, it could mean a lot of things. It could mean bad weather and they had to turn back, or . . ."

He interrupted me, "The weather here is good. It's windy, but you can see the mountaintops. The weather's good."

"So, it isn't weather. We've had no word. I worry they're in trouble. I hope they didn't crash."

"Sorry, Doctor. I hope they're okay. We'll do the best we can here. If they show up, we'll have them call you right away. Could you send us a ground ambulance, so we know help is on the way?"

The nurses recognized trouble with one look at my face. The secretary dispatched an ambulance to the lodge. I grabbed a phone book and, with some fumbling, found a number for Anchorage International Airport Air Traffic Control. After being transferred from location to location, I finally talked to a controller who connected me to the person handling flight following. "I hope you can help me. I'm Dr. Kelly McKay, medical control tonight for the helicopter program at Regional. I'm worried. Our helicopter left two hours ago and is overdue at Eureka Lodge. Any word on their position?"

"We can't track them in that area on radar at their low flight altitudes. They usually radio in when they depart our airspace. I'll check, but I don't think we had any communication from them this evening at all. Hold and I'll check with the others." He came back on line. "They confirm, no communication. What time did they take off?"

I looked at the secretary's notes. "The call came in from the Lodge at twenty-three forty-five. The ship lifted off within fifteen minutes."

The controller's voice came back. "I'll report them overdue and initiate a search. How many souls on board?"

"Three, the pilot and two medical personnel."

I hung up in shock.

Staff gathered around the desk.

"The ship never made it to Eureka Lodge. Air traffic control had no communication with them at all." I sat down, weak and in disbelief. "We have to presume the worst. It could be a precautionary landing in an area of radio blackout because of the mountains." My voice trembled. Tears welled. "Or, they crashed."

My thoughts raced, out of sync. I wasn't sure what to do.

The upset staff fired questions at me.

I tried to get them back to caring for the patients. "We won't know for a while. We have to keep working. If they crashed, it's seldom a structural problem with the aircraft. It's almost always pilot error." I asked the secretary to call the administrator to come in and help with decisions and then continued my explanation to the staff. "Crashing in bad weather with low visibility is the most frequent cause of fatal accidents. But the man I spoke with at the Lodge reported clear skies."

Inside, my gut twisted because of the ominous situation.

Nausea surged when I considered another cause. I didn't tell them, but Dale said he was tired. Could he have been too tired to fly?

Was he drinking out there in the call room?

Maybe Dale was flying drunk.

One of the nurses asked, "So, what do we do now?"

"We need to tend to what's going on here. The administrator is on his way in. I'll call the ER medical director to come in and handle everything else."

One nurse held back a sob. "What about Lynn?"

"I'm not sure. I guess the best thing is to let her sleep for now. Maybe we'll get some good news, and we can all stop worrying."

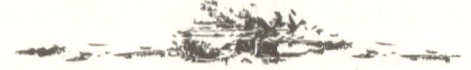

The administrator and ER director arrived. I thought I'd be able to pay attention to patient care, but my distraction showed. The ER director said, "Kelly, you look like you're dragging. If you'd like to go home and stay with Lynn, I'll cover. There is nothing we can do anyway except wait."

"If you'll take the new patients, I'll finish up the patients I've started. If they're down, I'm going out with the Civil Air Patrol to search."

The director checked the schedule. "Lynn is supposed to work in the morning. I'll find someone to cover for her."

"Thanks. Unless they find the ship on the ground waiting for help, Lynn won't be fit to work. Could you get coverage for both of us for two shifts? Then, we are off together for four days. We were going to do something fun."

News media would pick up the report on the overdue medical flight, so we had to tell the families of the three men on the helicopter before they heard it from friends or on the news. The ER medical director telephoned family members of the medical personnel on board. I heard voices talking on telephones at the desk making the dreaded calls. "Overdue, not crashed, but yes, I'm sorry. They're overdue."

I called the Civil Air Patrol at 3 a.m. and found Leo. The commander had called him in to man the radios and begin calling search pilots. I volunteered to fly after a nap. Leo said, "Go home and go to bed. The bad weather moved in and we're below flight minimums. No aircraft are in the air. I'll call when it's legal to fly. Better weather in the area of the search is forecast for mid-morning."

The storm struck with cold, gusty winds. Driving rain swept the city. It had been so balmy when I went to work the preceding evening I hadn't even worn a sweater. I walked out of the ER into pelting rain that drenched my clothes and plastered my hair to my head. I felt alive, glad to be alive, and forgot about all the warnings and phone calls. It didn't even cross my mind someone might follow me in this weather. By the time I got to the apartment, I was shivering uncontrollably. A hot shower and putting on a polar fleece jogging outfit with wool socks finally brought warmth.

The backlit clock on the stove showed three-thirty. I quietly opened the drapes covering the deck door and sat down at the adjacent table. Rain came down in sheets, dimming the outline of nearby homes. The spring sky was darker than usual, triggering the automated street lights to turn on. Tree limbs whipped about by the wind bent till they looked like they'd snap. The wind's roar muffled the sound of a metal garbage can lid careening down the alley in the wind. The disc rolled, went airborne, and bounced a couple times before striking a fence behind the apartment. Rain struck the deck door with force and pooled on the cement patio.

Should I wake Lynn? What could we do? We didn't know if Dale and the others were dead. All we could do was wait.

I went to the refrigerator. Inside, nothing looked edible. I poured a glass of milk and sat down at the table.

Lynn's door opened, pepper spray in hand. "Kelly, is that you? I think the storm woke me. Why are you home at this hour? Are you sick?"

I tried to hold back tears.

She studied my face.

"Kelly, what's wrong?" She walked toward me. Louder, she asked, "Kelly, what's wrong?"

I stood up and held her tight. "The helicopter is overdue."

"No. Oh, no, no. It can't be," she cried out in disbelief. "Dale's such a good pilot." She let out a gasp but no tears. "What happened?"

"They left for Eureka Lodge about midnight and never made it."

She peered out the window at the raging storm. "He flew in that?" She raised her voice, "He flew into a fucking storm and killed them all?"

"No, the weather hit long after they left. The weather in the direction of flight was good."

"Did they crash?" She shook me. "Tell me. Did they crash?"

"We don't know." I explained what had transpired.

Lynn finally cried. I stood with my arms around her, crying with her. Her thin body was racked with sobs. She asked more questions. "Did you see Dale?"

"No. He left when you were still there and didn't come back to the ER all evening. Rob talked to him by phone as usual after we got the call. Dale followed protocol and checked the weather just before they left."

"Oh, God, I hope he wasn't drinking." She cried louder.

"How could he? He was out in the hangar."

"I was out there recently to talk to him and opened their little refrigerator. There was a six-pack of O'Doul's. I asked him why."

"What'd he say?"

He became furious. "I like it. Do you have a problem?"

"Lynn, O'Doul's is non-alcoholic. It's okay if he drank that.

"Maybe he kept it there so if someone smelled alcohol on his breath he could use it as an excuse. He could show them he was just drinking O'Doul's."

"I plan to go on the search with CAP."

"You're not leaving me here. I'm going, too."

I explained that Leo would call.

"You go to bed. I'll wake you when he calls."

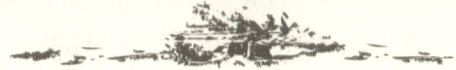

Lynn and I decided to go down to the CAP before Leo called. We couldn't stand waiting. I wasn't sure how she'd handle the situation and questioned her decision.

"Kelly, I have to be there. I have to help. If I'm doing something, it will be better than if I try to sit by the phone." She pulled on her jacket and handed me mine.

"Since I'm flying my plane, you can come as my observer. I couldn't take you in one of the CAP planes since you aren't a member."

We sat with Leo. His phone rang. He grunted a few words and hung up. "FAA says an airliner picked up an ELT signal out in the direction of their flight."

I gripped Lynn's arm. "Oh, no."

"I'm afraid so." His chubby face looked sad. "Dale is one of our best pilots."

Lynn asked, "What's an ELT? What's wrong?"

Leo turned away from his array of radios. "Emergency locator transmitter. It's a radio hardwired into aircraft, designed to only go off on impact, like a hard landing or a crash. A signal is transmitted, and other aircraft can home in on it and find the site it is coming from. It doesn't always mean a crash—turbulence or just bumpy air could trigger it. But because we know the chopper is overdue, we consider the worst when it's reported like this one."

I went outside and came back after looking at the sky. "The weather looks flyable here. How is it toward the east?"

"Weather is lifting in that area. I'll start calling pilots in."

"Let's go." I took Lynn's arm and pulled her out the door. We got back in my car and drove along the perimeter road to the other side of the airport and the Maule. The plane glistened bright yellow from the rain. Large puddles made it difficult to untie the ropes without getting wet.

Lynn struggled to remove the rope from the wing on the passenger side as I tugged on the other, unable to loosen it.

A body brushed my back and strong male hands reached over me and easily untied the knot. John Reilly, the CAP birdman, had emerged from the shadows to help. He smiled. "You were having a rough time, Dr. Mc Kay. Glad I could help."

His closeness and presence shocked me, but his beautiful, disarming smile was calming. Why was he at my plane?

"Where are you and your friend heading? Do you have room for another passenger?"

"Thanks for the help, John, but we're headed out on a search."

"I'm a good searcher." He stood forlorn, hands at his sides, fists clenched.

"I'm sorry, but I can't take you on this flight." He watched me finish the preflight and untie the tail rope.

Birdman stood under the wing of an adjacent plane and watched us taxi away.

We flew a pattern directed by Search Coordinator Leo. I tuned in the emergency channel and followed the Glenn Highway toward Eureka Lodge. The ominous high-pitched ELT drone got louder the closer we got to Chickaloon Pass.

Lynn followed our route on the map. "There's a large building down there on the side of the road. I think it's the Grizzly Roadhouse. We stopped in there on our snowmobile trip."

I flew at about a thousand feet. Mountains towered around us. Clouds engulfed the higher terrain, obscuring the peaks. Wind buffeted the plane. We flew past Sheep Mountain with the locator blaring. When we angled north around the mountain, the intensity decreased. I turned back and explained to Lynn, "The transmitter suddenly got less, which means we probably flew past it. We need to look around Sheep Mountain."

Her eyes widened. She didn't respond.

We circled down to about five hundred feet. "Airplanes on the ground are very difficult to see. If they're bright colors like this one, they stand out against the terrain better. Our chopper colors are maroon with white trim, which would be difficult to see. The snow is completely melted from the lower levels, so there is no contrast. Look for anything that doesn't look natural."

I flew a grid pattern for about half an hour. "I shouldn't have had so much coffee. My bladder is complaining."

"Me, too. Do we have to go back to Anchorage to go to the bathroom?"

"If we were guys, we could get out our little yellow bottles. Unfortunately, it's not as easy for a woman. Did you see the airstrip near the Roadhouse? We'll land there. Can I have the map for a minute?" She handed it to me.

I checked the runway details and set up for landing. Flying a left-hand pattern, first paralleling the runway and then turning the base leg, we flew at a low altitude. Just as I turned for landing, Lynn exclaimed, "Don't land. Don't land! Fly straight ahead. Look"

At about the 500-foot level, something didn't look right. We got closer. "I think you found them."

She cried out. "It's the helicopter. Kelly, oh, no, it's scattered in pieces. What I saw was broken trees and the skids. Circle lower."

"We can't go much lower. The winds are gusty. We have to think of our safety." I circled again and surveyed the site. "You're right, Lynn. Wreckage is strewn, broken in two major pieces with the tail boom separated. I'll get the exact coordinates from the GPS. It will only take a minute, and then we'll go to the Roadhouse and call Anchorage on their landline."

She pushed her microphone away from her mouth and bowed her head. Her body shook as she cried.

I tried to pay attention to landing. "We can hike up to the crash site. It isn't very far off the road."

Chapter 27 A Fatal Mistake

We landed at the Roadhouse airstrip and called flight coordination to report the crash site. By the time a ground team prepared to hike to the site arrived, Lynn and I had calmed our emotions, but the men did not want us along. The thought of seeing bodies of friends mangled in wreckage brought a flood of memories of my injuries and the plane crash that killed my father, but, like Lynn, I had to go.

"I need to see for myself. I'm going." Lynn stiffened, with fists clenched and tears streaming. Her stomping steps echoed from the wooden floor, and the heavy door slammed behind her.

Four men and I followed. Lynn slowed, allowing them to precede us across the highway and into the treed incline. "What happens now? Will the search team remove the bodies?"

"More people will be arriving to help with that. NTSB and the FAA will go over the wreckage looking for mechanical causes."

Lynn climbed faster than I did but then sat on a boulder, giving me time to catch my breath after a scramble over a scree field. "I told Dale I wouldn't marry him if he continued to drink."

"Do you think he was flying drunk?"

"I never thought he would, but I don't know."

"On autopsies, they always check for drugs and alcohol. Cornell Ramsey will likely be doing the postmortems on all of them."

"I hope Dale didn't kill two innocent people. Rob suspected him of drinking before flying second seat on a fixed-wing flight. Now they're both dead along with the flight medic."

The mile climb to the crash site left me exhausted. Physically, Lynn was stronger, but we were both emotional wrecks. The men had split up and were scouring the area.

Lynn and I scanned the debris field. We walked to the main fuselage. A uniformed body strapped in the pilot's seat hung motionless, his head twisted, helmet ajar. The hair was unmistakably Dale's. The features were not recognizable due to bloody crush injuries.

Lynn reached in and softly touched his face. Her fingers pulled back as if she had contacted a hot stove.

I put my arm around her. "Let's go."

An older man at my side stepped back after looking inside the cracked fuselage and in the tail section yards away. "It was a rapid, violent end for all of them. They died on impact."

We left the men behind to secure the site until the authorities arrived. We made our way down the slope to the airstrip.

Lynn's words were hard, resigned. "This certainly changes things for all of us. I can't believe this happened. Dale's father is old. He'll take it hard."

"It's devastating to the flight program. We've lost three of the flight team, including the chief pilot. The public loss of confidence will take a long time to repair, if ever, especially if Dale was drunk."

Chapter 28 Grief

Wailing, funerals, and a temporary closure of the helicopter flight program were a destructive force within the once-cohesive emergency room staff. Dr. Ramsey called me a few days after the accident with condolences. "Kelly, I wanted you and Lynn to know before it came out in tomorrow's paper. Dale's blood alcohol was elevated, in fact, was high. He was legally drunk."

I felt weak and sat down. "Terrible news. Drunk. Flying drunk. Thank you for telling us in advance of the public report. Lynn will take it hard."

"Unfortunately, he took the other two down with him. A real tragedy. Based on NTSB's report, the impact was uncontrolled. Not related to engine issues and a hard autorotation landing. Not much left of any of the bodies. How is Lynn holding up?"

"Not talking much. Still at the disbelief stage. We have the funerals out of the way, and I have encouraged her to go right back to work. Try to keep busy."

"It's usually best to do that. Let me know if I can help."

"With the report of Dale's blood alcohol, it will be more difficult for her to face the staff knowing he was at fault. They were engaged to be married."

"She isn't responsible for his actions. They'll know, but it's a tough situation for everyone."

I thanked him again and hung up, wondering how Lynn would take the news.

Lynn's bedroom door opened. "Who called?"

"Cornell Ramsey. Bad news. Dale was legally drunk."

Lynn shrieked and sat at the kitchen table. "That dumb son of a bitch! Why did he have to kill two wonderful people? I killed Rob. I killed Rob and the EMT just as much as Dale did. I should have turned him in. I hate myself."

"Lynn don't be silly. You tried. You never saw him drink on the job or while he was flying, did you?"

"No, but the thought crossed my mind when I saw that O'Doul's in his work refrigerator. I believed in him. I trusted him. He was very intelligent and could be such a nice man. I will miss him so much." She took a deep irregular breath, trying to stifle a sob.

"We have another day off. Let's go for a drive. Or, would you rather go for a flight?" I asked hesitantly.

"I want to fly. Maybe it will help ease my conscience and gloom. I want to fly over the crash site again."

"Are you sure?"

"It might help. Flying over the site may help to finalize it for me. It's hard to let go. I'm glad we went to the crash so I could see his body. I shipped that urn of ashes off to his father. What a terrible end."

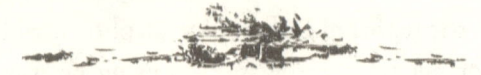

Near Anchorage, white clouds hung in the sky like puffs of cotton. The air got bumpy above the highway as it wandered along a pass between scenic mountain peaks and along the Matanuska River. We watched for Sheep Mountain. As we neared, we both saw the crash site location.

The debris and aircraft pieces had been removed, leaving only a few broken trees to mark the spot. It was difficult to tell anything bad had happened there.

I circled lower.

"The dumb shit flew right into a fucking mountain and killed himself. It's as simple as that. Smart man, but dumb, very dumb." Lynn slumped. "Kelly, let's fly over to Susitna. You don't have to land but show me up close why you loved it so much. I need to see something to make me happy."

I landed on Susitna just like Marty taught me. I touched down just to the right of the white jug.

Lynn and I sat on rocky ground on the mountaintop. We cried and laughed and cried some more. The view, the fresh air, and the escape were therapeutic. I got up and pulled her to her feet. "I haven't eaten much in days. I'm finally feeling hungry. Let's go to the Captain Cook and have a good meal."

The delicious gourmet food filled us. We didn't drink.

At home, the answering machine's red light blinked. Two messages. I pushed the button, dreading who it might be. The first one was Marty with condolences; he had talked to Dr. Ramsey. The second caller had hung up without leaving a message.

Chapter 29 Too Close

After my next day shift, I drove to Merrill and practiced pattern work, doing many takeoffs and landings before flying westward across the inlet in a breeze off the salt water. The sun dipped below the horizon like as sinking red ball that turning the sky orange. Thin layers of purple clouds disappeared with the sun. I didn't want to go home, but by the time I landed, my stomach told me to eat.

Sleep came easy after eating Chinese takeout and the stress release of flying. The morning radio alarm pulled me slowly from sleep, leaving little time to get ready for work. I took a rapid hot shower, shoved a bagel in my pocket, and, with wet hair and wearing a polar fleece jacket, I unlocked the deadbolt to leave.

I pushed on the door. I couldn't open it. There was pressure against it, as if someone was playing a trick and blocking me inside. My heart rate increased. "Who's out there?"

No answer.

I pushed again and still met with resistance. It moved a little and then closed again, as if something was wedged against the door.

I pushed hard with my shoulder. More success. I squeezed one foot out on the step and nudged the door enough to get my head and shoulder partway between the door and its frame. Something heavy struck my foot. I looked down and screamed.

A hand. A body.

I tried to jump back but was wedged in place. Until I pushed against the door, not to squeeze out but to get back inside, I was caught looking down at the corpse of a young woman.

The body toppled over onto the landing with a dull thud when I could finally move the door. She'd been somehow propped against the door. The mottled white and purple hand with broken scarlet acrylic nails appeared to be grasping for the railing.

Torn clothing partially covered her M-shaped thigh laceration that was leaking dark blood onto the entryway.

I backed into the apartment, closed and locked the door, and dialed 9-1-1.

I waited for the ambulance with my handgun on the table, listening.

The silent neighborhood provided no clues. No movement. I checked the deck door and found it secured.

The windows were locked. I peeked through a slit in the drapes and saw no one.

I hoped no one would see the body, stiff with rigor mortis, lying on my door step.

Sirens edged closer, reducing my anxiety.

The phone rang. Its ring startled me. I let the answering machine answer. "Kelly are you there? Kelly, answer me, Kelly. Oh, my God." The voice wailed, "She doesn't answer."

Lynn.

I switched off the machine. "Lynn, it's okay. I'm here. I'm all right."

"Oh, Kelly," Lynn sobbed. "We heard the ambulance dispatched to our address for a woman down. Possible ten-sixty. I thought he got you."

"I have to go. There's an officer pounding on the deck door. When I was leaving for work, I found a dead woman at our front door. I'll be late for work."

"I'll be here. You can bet I'm not coming home."

Chapter 30 Another Murder

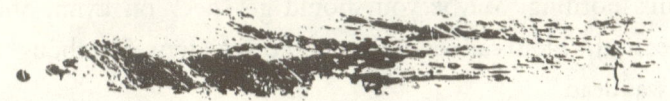

I opened my front window drapes to see an ambulance with lights still flashing blocking the street directly in front. Uniformed officers cordoned off a crowd of gathering neighbors, gawkers, and news media. Dr. Ramsey appeared in the crowd soon after Rick Moore and Virgil Wescott had wrapped yellow plastic crime scene tape across the front of the apartment building.

The picture evolved like a movie; I wished it wasn't real.

Medics huddled with officers and then disappeared around the side of the apartment building. I heard a knock on the deck door and pulled back the drape to find two of my medic friends, part of my team. I opened the door. "Hi. Come in."

One big guy entered behind a petite medic with a bouncy ponytail and enviable biceps. She had to be strong mentally and physically to perform the rigorous job beside the big dudes. "Dr. McKay, you've had a lot of badness following you around lately. Bob and I had nothing to do out front. We came to check on you. Are you okay?"

"I'm all right, I guess, especially since it's not me out there dead on the step."

"Where's Lynn?"

"At work doing my day shift after working all night. I found that poor woman when I was trying to leave for work this morning. Maybe you should go check on Lynn. She heard the radio call sending you to this address. She thought I was dead."

"Do you know that woman?"

"I didn't get a good look at her face, but knew she was dead. I locked the door and called 9-1-1."

"Did you hear anything?"

"It was the best night's sleep I've had since the helicopter went down. I didn't hear a thing."

"I wonder if she was trying to get help. If you're sure you are all right, we'll stop by the hospital and talk to Lynn."

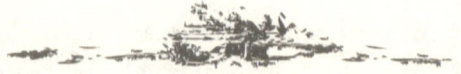

I made a large pot of very strong coffee, poured myself a mug, and sat at the table still wearing my bright green polar fleece. I felt cold and worried and definitely did not want to go outside to look at another body. Footsteps and a knock brought my attention to the deck door, where Dr. Ramsey stood with Detectives Moore and Wescott.

I motioned them to come in. Ramsey sat beside me. "Kelly, this isn't good. We're all very concerned. I took a look at the victim. Her injuries are the same as the other two. It's a serial killer."

The detectives fired questions at me. "Did you hear any noise or commotion last night?"

"Nothing. After an evening flight alone, I went to bed about eleven and slept all night. Best night's sleep in a long time." I told them about trying to leave for work and how I found her body. "Do you think she tried to get away from somebody and died on my step?"

"No, Kelly. She has drag marks. She died somewhere else and was placed at your door, just like Misty on Crow Creek Pass Trail."

Rick cut in. "We talked outside before coming in to discuss this with you. Your life is obviously at risk."

"She was strangled. She also has a large laceration on her thigh, just like the others," Clark said. "It's his signature. Kelly, you've seen all three. We think he's trying to tell you something."

"He's getting closer and closer," Virgil stressed. "This is not a coincidence. He's getting bold. You could be next."

"I think you need to leave Anchorage, and Lynn too. The hospital won't be too happy with two of their favorite doctors running off, but it's temporary until we get the bastard. I have an arrest warrant out for your old surgeon friend, Brett Warren."

Cornell wanted to know, "Do you have a place to go to hide out for a while?"

"I suppose we could visit our parents."

"Seattle is not a good option if it's the surgeon. That's what he'd expect you to do, and he might be able to find you."

"I don't like running. I don't want to leave Alaska. Couldn't we just fly somewhere? Lynn and I were planning to go to Hot Dam Hot Springs in a couple weeks. That's far away." Cornell nodded. "We don't have to tell anyone where we are going. Besides, I don't think the other ER docs can cover us with no warning."

Cornell pulled out his cell phone. "This isn't a choice. It's critical. I'll call the administrator. He'll take care of it."

"Isn't it too early to be calling him? I doubt if he comes in before nine."

"He's my brother-in-law. Damn it, I'll get him out of bed." I'd never heard Cornell raise his voice before. He called, explained the circumstances, and hung up. About ten minutes later, Cornell's phone rang. "I knew you could do it. We'll send a car over to ER to pick up Lynn."

He hung up. "The ER physician director is on his way in and will cover today and revamp the schedule while you are both away."

Virgil looked out the front drapes. "There is still a crowd out front. Start packing for both of you, Kelly. We'll have an unmarked car come up the alley to pick you both up. You're leaving town right now. We need to be sure you're safe, so we can devote our efforts to finding him.

They asked more questions. I had few answers.

Lynn swung in the back door accompanied by an officer. "What a snarled mess out there. Now what are we going to do?" She came over and hugged me so tight I couldn't breathe.

"We are leaving town. Throw a few changes of clothes in a pack."

"Where are we going?"

"To Hot Dam, a little earlier than planned."

A car pulled up in the alley.

Virgil said, "I've been to Hot Dam. It's at the edge of the earth, and that's far enough. You'll be safe. Bring your swimsuits and mosquito repellant."

The officer that had brought Lynn in walked us out to the waiting car. The driver delivered us to the plane and helped pull it from the parking place. Lynn lifted the gull-wing door and slid in. She latched the door while I did the walk-around, checking everything. I thanked the officer. He stood by and watched as I checked the oil and finished the walk-around.

I taxied into position and held for takeoff. After a short wait with two other aircraft ahead of us in line, the tower cleared us to the active runway. "November Nine One One Delta Romeo, pull into position and hold for departing aircraft." A Lake Amphibian climbed out ahead of us and turned. "November Nine One One Delta Romeo, you are cleared for takeoff. Please state your intentions."

"One Delta Romeo, straight-out departure, then north when able."

"What is your destination?"

I stumbled, not wanting to say where we were going. "Circle, I guess, Circle."

Left turnout approved. Have a good flight."

"One Delta Romeo."

With liftoff, I had a feeling of relief. Not only were we out of acute danger from some madman, but we were flying. Flying was much safer than being on the ground. Initially, we climbed toward the Chugach Range. The morning, sun filtered by thin clouds, brightened the irregular ridgeline. When we turned north, a sudden feeling of anger swept over me. "I'm damn mad. I really like this area and feel like a child being sent away by a parent for something I didn't do, like I've been bad. I don't want to go."

Lynn shook her head. "No. It's kind of a forced vacation, but we need to get away. I had trouble getting through last night. The staff is so depressed. Even Vic, who survived hazardous military time and saw a lot of badness, talked about finding a different line of work."

"We'd really have trouble if he left. It is great working with him. He said Rob's wife is pregnant with their first child."

An emptiness lingered until Merrill Field Tower interrupted my dark thoughts. "You are now leaving our control area. Frequency change approved."

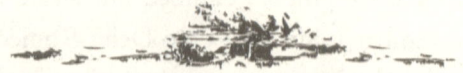

I followed the highway toward Eagle River, avoiding the restricted areas around Elmendorf Air Force Base and Fort Richardson. After crossing Knik Arm, the tidal water stretching inland toward Matanuska Glacier, we followed the Parks Highway. From 8,000 feet, we saw the narrow black ribbon snaking northward, with toy cars and campers in long lines moving in both directions.

Lynn peered down. "Look at all those poor bastards in traffic. Reminds me of being in Boston surrounded by people. Fenced in. I'll never go back. Alaska is wide open and wonderful."

"Based on how slow the cars are moving down there, I think we'll be in Fairbanks before they make it to Denali. Flying simplifies getting from one place to another."

I circled Marty's house near the Talkeetna airport. One of his planes was gone, so we didn't land for a visit. Continuing north, we hit turbulence flying through Windy Pass with up- and downdrafts severe enough that one bump whacked my head on the side window. I reduced power to ride out the turbulence.

Lynn cinched her belt tighter. "I'll be glad to get back to smooth air again, but I always did like carnival rides!"

"Marty had me fly this route through Windy Pass a number of times. Some pilots get confused here. The pass is only twenty miles long, but it has a couple of narrow spots. In bad weather, some flatlanders have turned after the first narrow area and ended up lost or dead."

"In spite of your horror stories, I feel pretty safe. But where is Circle? Aren't we going to Hot Dam Hot Springs?"

I explained that Circle is close to Hot Dam and that I didn't want to announce to the world where we were headed.

Lynn and I bantered back and forth during the flight. Her delicate features relaxed. Her curly blond hair fluffed around her face like a little girl's. Her blue eyes were bright, but when she lapsed into silence, I sensed the grief she was trying to hide.

Chapter 31 Hot Dam Escape

Let me know when you see Fairbanks. I know where it's supposed to be, based on our GPS, but I still don't see it. We'll refuel there." I kept looking for the sprawling city, which was difficult to pick out against the flat tundra horizon. "Satellite navigation makes flying easy. You can know exactly where you are and still be lost."

Lynn scanned. "That gives me confidence."

We both spotted Fairbanks, and I radioed Approach Control for Fairbanks International when we were about ten miles out. The controller cleared me for a straight-in approach to the north/south runway.

As the city came into better view, we looked for the airport. "I've never landed here before. I saw on a map the runway parallels a lake that is a controlled airport for seaplanes, like Lake Spenard is in Anchorage. It's more difficult to set up for landing straight in when you can't find the airport." I reduced power to descend.

Lynn pointed off in the distance. "I see it, now. The airport looks big, but it sure was difficult to make out. Now that I know where to look, it's obvious."

Upon landing, Ground Control directed us to the fixed-base operator for fuel. I asked the man next door at Flight Service for information about Hot Dam.

He pointed to a map on the wall. "It's about a one-hundred-fifty-mile flight from Fairbanks. VFR was not recommended one hour ago, but weather is improving. Forecast now is for broken 1,500, overcast 3,000. Very do-able. By the time you get there, it may be better. Take a look. Come on back if you don't like it."

Lynn asked, "Could we call the hotel for reservations? We want to stay a few days."

The man chuckled. "They have HF radiotelephone, but it's not reliable. They'll let you sleep in the lobby until a room opens up. It's quite a place and worth the trip. Even home cooking. Vegetables from the garden watered from the springs."

Lynn looked at me aghast. "What are you getting us into?"

The terrain remained relatively flat along our northeast route, but because of low visibility we had to sneak over a ridge just beneath a cloud layer to proceed. Once over the high spot near Circle, visibility improved enough to keep going. Below us, the harsh, desolate landscape showed little evidence of habitation other than a few placer mines. A narrow dirt road carried few cars and an occasional tour bus.

After a low-altitude circle over the area to survey the airport and hotel, we landed on the gravel runway in a heavy mist. As soon as the prop stopped, our windows turned gray with mosquitoes. We rushed to push the plane onto a grassy area with waiting tie-down ropes.

Mosquitoes swarmed in high-pitched humming clouds, flying in my eyes and mouth and up my nose. I yanked up my hood and tied it shut with a few trapped inside. "These mosquitoes are killers. Let's get the heck out of here."

Lynn hoisted our two small backpacks out of the baggage compartment. "These have the essentials. We can come back later for the rest of our stuff."

I looped ropes through rings on the wings and tail and then tied them to the ground rings. Lynn ran along the quarter-mile dirt road toward the hotel with me close on her heels. I lost sight of her when she turned a corner and disappeared from view, along the scrub pine lined road.

The relentless mosquitoes followed us. When I caught up with Lynn, the backs of her pants legs were fuzzy with a moving layer of bloodsuckers. We ran into the lobby of the old four-story structure as if fleeing killer bees.

A teenage boy looked up from his book when we burst in. He placed his book out of view. "Trying to outrun the bugs?" He smiled as we approached. Our footsteps echoed off scarred wooden floors partially hidden beneath large, strategically placed, flowered carpets. Overstuffed couches and chairs lined the perimeter of the large foyer.

"Hello, ladies. Welcome to Hot Dam. Do you have reservations?"

"No. We made the decision to come in a hurry. Do you have any rooms?"

"I have a couple. One with two doubles, the other with a queen."

Lynn dropped the packs and pulled out a credit card. "We'll take the two doubles."

"How long you planning to stay?"

We looked at each other. I shrugged. "We aren't sure."

"First come, first served. You can stay as long as you like. Sometimes people don't show up, or they get here and the lack of facilities or the mosquitoes scare them away. We call it a real Alaskan experience. I hope you like it here." He had us sign the register. "Where you from?"

"We just flew in from Fairbanks."

"I heard you fly over, so I knew someone would be coming in." He pointed to a swinging door. "There's a small hotel bar on the end by the pools. Everything is open twenty-four hours a day. The sun doesn't go down this far north. It confuses people trying to keep track of mealtimes. We serve each meal for a two-hour period, and there's always coffee on."

The young man led us up three flights of noisy, uncarpeted stairs, where he proudly opened the door and handed us each a skeleton key. "You are probably too young to have ever used one of these."

Lynn examined her key. "I've seen them in secondhand stores in boxes, but I've never opened a door with one."

"It's not a secure lock, but we've never had trouble around here except with rowdy drunks. If you have anything valuable, keep it with you, or I can put it in the safe."

He started to walk away, but then he turned and cautioned, "The food is good, the men are friendly, the liquor is strong, and the pools are hot. Be careful." He hesitated. "I think I should warn you, the miners come in some nights. They're heavy drinkers and will hit on you, so beware."

Lynn thanked him and pushed open the door. "I think he is too young to be telling us these things, but it sounds like he's been doing his job for a while."

I walked in and sat in a straight-backed chair near the only window in our room. "This is the kind of hotel I remember seeing in old western movies." Iron frames supported two double-sized mattresses covered with white chenille bedspreads. "My grandmother had a bedspread like this with a few tufts missing. I haven't seen one in twenty years. Have you?"

Lynn threw herself on a bed. "Nope. Never have. Cool. This is a cool place. No frills." She rolled back and forth, springs squeaking with each roll. "This is definitely the place to bring my folks. My mother will think I've lost my mind." Lynn changed her voice. "My dear Lynn, would you call the concierge?" Lynn roared.

A narrow dresser on bowed legs stood alone against one wall, with an oval mirror with a peeling silver coating on the back hanging above. Near a small table crowded by two wooden chairs stood an ancient floor lamp with a fringed shade. A line drawing of a polar bear looked down on us.

Lynn sat up. "I bet you could use a drink after all your flying. I hate to mention drinking, but we don't have issues like Dale. Sorry I mentioned his name. I wasn't going to do that."

We put on swimsuits beneath our pants and T-shirts and stuffed our wallets in our pockets before walking downstairs to check out the bar and pools.

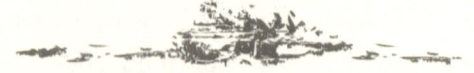

We joined a few restless afternoon drinkers sitting along a bar lined with flickering jar candles inside a dark room smelling of old beer. After one expensive icy brew, we left to experience the hot springs.

In cool air, we ran along a narrow trail swarming with mosquitoes and entered a large building covered with weathered, translucent, corrugated fiberglass. The hot steamy air tickled my nose and sent me into a coughing spasm while I tried to read the extensive instructions about the proper use of the many pools.

Signs near each pool carried warnings, temperatures, and recommended time limits depending on your health and heat tolerance. I chose to go from cooler to warmer and adjust slowly to each change. Lynn decided to alternate hot and cold. My skin turned white and wrinkly within an hour. Lynn looked at her skin and laughed. "I think we melted our body fat in that hot pool. It's definitely time to get out, and I'm starved."

We went to dinner in blue jeans and joined eight others at a long table. A New York couple named Barb and Ray kept us laughing for an hour. Barb liked Hot Dam, and Ray was in television withdrawal. "I can't believe I actually let her drag me here. I don't hike—I don't want to waste any heartbeats with exercise. We're only given so many, and I spend mine frugally. My thumb is itching for a TV channel changer."

Lynn and I talked about the healthy food. Ray rolled his eyes. "I can't believe you ladies think this is food. Barb is trying to kill me. I haven't had a french fry in a week."

Delicious bowls of vegetables and platters of fried chicken were passed around the table, enough to feed twice as many people. Ray ate more than his share.

The perky waitress in blue jeans and a T-shirt, wearing a little apron, talked directly to Ray. "You should take these good-looking women on a hike to an area where you can see the old dam this place is named for. "It's an easy trail. Everybody who comes here does it, even the old ones."

Ray looked forlorn, "How about the old, slow ones?"

She tried to shame him into it. "Them, too. It's pretty flat. If an eighty-year-old granny can do it, you can. It's worth the walk."

Lynn and I decided to go out to the airplane to get our other packs. Barb talked Ray into walking to the airplane with us. "I'll do it if you don't make me run. Do either of you know CPR?"

We laughed. Lynn said, "We are both ER doctors."

"Well then, let me change my question. Can you ream out my arteries if they decide to snap shut out here on the tundra?"

Barb elbowed his fat arm. "No, so you better behave."

"Well, heck. Two good-lookin' women pumping on my chest and giving me mouth-to-mouth would be just fine with me."

At 9 p.m. north of the Arctic Circle, the sun drilled holes in the cloud layer and a brisk wind thinned the mosquitoes. The four of us first walked to the dam site and then out to the airplane. Ray scoffed when he saw the plane. "You don't really get in that thing, now do you ladies?"

"Tomorrow, I'll take both of you for a scenic flight, if you are interested."

Barb sounded excited. "Yes, yes, yes. We'll go!"

Ray muttered, "No one ever told me what I'd have to put up with, married to you. Will you hold my hand if I get scared?"

I think he was serious. She agreed to hold his hand.

Lynn laughed. "Ray, Kelly carries a box of Ziploc bags in a seat back. It's a barf bag if you get air sick. I'll hand you a bag, but I'm not holding your hand."

He held back and looked at the three of us. "I like being with women, but how was I unlucky enough to get stuck with three tough broads like you?"

We laughed over another beer, and in the midnight daylight, we climbed the three flights to our room. I locked the door and put a chair in front of it.

"Being cautious, huh? Where's your pepper spray? Where's your gun? I've had my pepper spray with me all day."

"I haven't been that good. My small canister is in the outside pocket of my pack. I'll put it in the pocket of my jeans by my bed right now so I don't forget. My gun is in the plane where I always keep it as part of survival gear."

"That's not a very good place for it, Kelly."

"Gosh. I have been having so much fun, I'd forgotten why we came here."

"I haven't."

Chapter 32 Survival

Footsteps running up the wooden stairs, followed by pounding on our door, alerted us to trouble. "Wake up. Wake up. We need help! There's been an accident. Can you fly someone to Fairbanks?"

"Just a minute." I got out of bed and moved the chair.

Lynn jumped from her bed and put her back to the door. She whispered, "Don't open the door."

I called. "Who's there? What happened?"

"It's Paul from the front desk. Some miners on their way home came upon a rollover. They brought a guy in here in bad shape."

"What time is it?"

"Four a.m."

"We'll get dressed and be down in a minute."

Lynn flipped on a light. "I don't like this, Kelly. We don't even have a stethoscope. I don't like being so far from help."

Paul waited outside the door. He took the steps down two at a time. We ran behind him to the lobby and out to the front of the hotel.

In the back of a pickup truck, an unconscious young man lay on a wooden door. The victim's legs were stiff. Periodically, he coughed. His arms stiffened. His back arched.

Another young man held the victim's head, trying to reduce movement.

After one look, I said to Lynn, "He's decerebrate. Needs a tube and a neurosurgeon, not us."

Paul looked over our shoulders, worried. "All we have is a first aid kit with some Band-Aids."

Lynn asked, "What happened?"

The young man holding the victim's head in alignment said, "We were heading back to the mine after a few beers here and found this guy lying in the road next to a car on its top. The other guy was dead."

Lynn climbed into the back of the truck to check the injured man. I surveyed the man on the door and the man holding the injured guy's head. "It looks like you are doing everything right. Are you medically trained?"

"I'm a paramedic from Kentucky working at the mine this summer. We have no medical gear."

"I'm glad you could start the basics. Here we are, two ER docs and a paramedic without their gear." Lynn knelt beside the injured man, feeling his head, neck, and chest, looking for injuries. "He's breathing all right now, but I wish we could tube him to protect his airway. Have you seen any meaningful movement, or has it always been this decerebrate posturing?"

He looked at both of us, relieved. "Just posturing. God, I'm glad you're here. I was feeling very lonely."

Lynn jumped out of the pickup. "We're glad you're here. The door was a great idea."

Paul backed away. "I'll prop the door open if you want to bring him in." He wedged the door open with a chair and then disappeared inside.

A miner needled the medic. "Yeah, Curtis, and now we got an outhouse without a door."

"We'll get it back. He's only borrowing it."

I went inside and found Paul fiddling with a radio. "We need a medical helicopter from Fairbanks." The sleepy young man said nervously, "I'm sorry, ma'am, but the radiophone is down. We don't have any way to get ahold of outside help. Besides, they don't have a medical helicopter in Fairbanks."

"Shit. That makes this a lot more complicated. Can you wake up a couple more guests to help us carry the guy in here? How about Barb and Ray from New York?"

Paul ran up the stairs and pounded on some doors. He returned looking pale. "My father will be here in a minute. He says there's a medical helicopter at the airbase that had to come out once last year."

Barb and Ray adjusted their clothes as they ran down the steps behind Paul's father. With six people helping, we lifted the makeshift backboard and carried the injured man inside to the lobby floor. Curtis held the patient's head, keeping his airway open, while Lynn and I checked for other injuries. No tools. No stethoscope made it easy. We looked and felt for injuries.

Someone handed me a penlight. The young man's pupils were equal but unreactive. Blood and fluid dripped from one ear.

Lynn reported, "His pulse is strong."

I pulled up his shirt and put my ear against his chest. "Wouldn't Osler be proud of me now? His lungs sound okay, moving air on both sides, and there's no big heart murmur."

Lynn and the medic sat on the floor, looking at the injured guy and then at each other. "I just talked to Paul. You won't believe this. There is no way to call out. They use a radio telephone system of some kind, and it's not working."

"Great," Curtis muttered. "Rural medicine at its best. I like having a chopper at hand to come in and bail us out. Just a radio call away in the city." Lynn and I agreed.

Paul listened. "Didn't some of you fly in? Can't you stick him in the back and fly him out?"

Lynn's sleepy eyes looked at me. "Can we?"

I shook my head, "There is no way we can fit him in the Maule even if we took the back seats out."

Curtis looked for another miner. "I could have one of the guys go back and use our radiophone at the mine. It doesn't work half the time, but they might be able to raise somebody to get help. The mine is thirty-five miles away."

I went to the door and looked at the weather. "I have an idea that might be faster. If there is a break in the clouds, I could fly up through it and get high enough to contact Fairbanks on the radio. They could then contact the air base and send help."

Lynn jumped up. "Do it. Can I get your keys or give you a hand?"

"I have the key in my pocket but could use some help. You take over here, Curtis . . ."

"Call me Curt."

"I'll get airborne. Map, radio frequencies, everything I need is in the plane."

Ray and Barb moved closer, worried. "What are you going to do?"

I explained as they followed me outside."

Ray looked up at the overcast. "Can you fly in these clouds?"

"I see a few holes developing in the cloud layer. Pilots call them sucker holes."

Now Barb sounded worried. "What do you mean by that?"

"They're called sucker holes because suckers fly up through them to get above the terrain and clouds. If the hole closes over, the sucker gets stuck above the clouds. It's fine if you have lots of gas and know you can see the ground where you are headed. The real problem is running low on gas and being lost above or in the clouds."

Ray shook his head. "Too chancy. You shouldn't go."

"There are some large breaks west of here. I should have no problem coming back if I can get back under the layer. I just hope I can raise Fairbanks on the radio. We're a long way from there."

The four of us trotted out to the plane. They helped untie the ropes and stepped back.

The engine started on the first try. I quickly taxied toward the end of the 3,500-foot gravel strip and pushed in full throttle. As the plane accelerated, various scenarios ran through my thoughts. Some of them were ominous, but we might be able to save a life if we could get the injured man transported to a high level of care.

I lifted off in just a few feet. I had set the GPS to Hot Dam for our flight in, so I had the coordinates for my return. If the sucker hole closed, I decided to circle down through the clouds right over the runway where there was no obstruction. This was not a legal maneuver for flying in clouds but possibly lifesaving for me under the circumstances.

If I didn't break out of the clouds at a safe height, based on the altimeter, I could climb back above the layer and head to Fairbanks or some other airstrip that might become visible along the route.

I could always land on the road.

There were lots of outs.

Once at a safe altitude, I kept climbing toward a hole in the overcast and tuned my radio to 121.5, the international emergency frequency. With the plane trimmed to its best climb speed, I circled up through the biggest hole, trying to remain clear of clouds. Wisps of thin clouds covered the plane. I could usually see through them. Soon I climbed into clear skies and bright sun, with the gray layer below like an unstable ocean surface. I circled up to 10,000 feet, periodically calling, "Fairbanks Radio, this is Maule November Nine One One Delta Romeo. Do you read?"

Silence.

Eleven thousand feet. Much higher, and I'd need oxygen. I had no oxygen available, so I would have to abort the effort.

After many discouraging calls with no response, I tried once again, "Fairbanks Radio, this is Maule November Nine One One Delta Romeo. Do you read me?"

"Aircraft calling Fairbanks, this is JAL Flight 197, can we help?" said a wonderfully accented voice.

"JAL, this is Maule One Delta Romeo circling over Hot Dam Hot Springs. Could you relay a message to Fairbanks Radio for me?"

"We'll give it a try. Go ahead."

"There has been a car accident near the hot springs. One killed and one critically injured. We need them to send a medical helicopter to Hot Dam Hot Springs Hotel."

I continued to circle and listen.

Finally, "Miss pilot calling JAL, please respond."

"This is Maule One Delta Romeo."

"We have confirmed a medical helicopter from Eielson Air Force Base will lift off soon. Estimated time to Hot Dam is two hours."

"JAL, thank you very much. One Delta Romeo."

"One Delta Romeo, you are welcome. Good luck."

After all my circling, I'd drifted fifteen miles north of Hot Dam. I circled lower but remained above the broken cloud layer until I neared the airstrip. Thankfully, dissipating clouds revealed large patches of ground, patches of tundra that all looked alike.

Without the GPS, I'd be totally lost in desolate country.

My heart pounded.

I'd accomplished what I set out to do. The weather cooperated. The helicopter would be here to help.

My legs felt weak, and my feet trembled as they controlled the rudder pedals. I circled lower and broke out below the clouds a couple of miles from the hotel airstrip. I landed and taxied to parking. Leaving the plane untied, I ran to the hotel with the good news.

Lynn sat holding the injured man's head.

Curt was asleep on the floor beside her.

Across the lobby, stretched out on a couch, an old miner and his dog snored.

The slam of the screen door awakened Curt.

Lynn looked at me. "How did it go?"

I gave them a thumb up. "A helicopter will be here in about ninety minutes."

Curt took over holding the man's neck in alignment. Lynn got up. "I was worried. Did you have trouble contacting them?"

I explained what had happened. "Are you tired? I could watch him for a while. My adrenaline is too high to sleep. Have you had any trouble with his airway?"

"Airway's fine. Hasn't vomited or aspirated. Pupils are equal, but he is moving less. That may be a bad sign." Lynn stretched her back and clenched and unclenched her fists, encouraging blood flow in her fingers. "I'm fine. Curtis did all the work. I just sat and talked to him until a few minutes ago. I think I put him to sleep."

"I wasn't sleeping but close to it. This has been a long night after a very long day mining gold. I'm not used to all this daylight." Curtis sat up. "I feel more energetic in Alaska than back in Kentucky. I just wish I could snore like the old miner George and his dog Color. They both got drunk earlier in the night. They're regulars here, maybe both alcoholic. They like their beer."

The patient coughed and stiffened his limbs. Curt watched the man's breathing.

Lynn said with hope, "The helicopter will have drugs and probably a doctor."

Curt stretched his arms. "I've had enough tubes. That's why I'm mining, just to get away from the street. I might go back someday."

I smiled at him. "You couldn't escape. Here you are using your skills in the wilds of Alaska."

"My dad's a doctor. He tried his best to get me interested in medical school. From the time we could walk, he brought me and my sister to the hospital to do rounds. I really wounded him when I was in grade school. He told a story of spending hours with me making rounds and looking at X-rays. He asked if I found it interesting. I told him I had a lot more fun touring the pizza parlor the preceding day and wanted to be one of those guys who tossed the pizza dough."

We laughed. "Neither Kelly nor I have doctors in our families. My family tried to make me a banker. I just wasn't cut out for it." Lynn added, "You may not be cut out for medicine, but the field you chose is just as challenging."

We sat on the floor in an exhausted trio around the injured man. I spun around after a firm tap on my shoulder and found myself looking straight at two large knees. A gargantuan male, over six feet tall, around age fifty and tilting the scales at about 350 pounds, stood behind me. Past his knees, I saw Ray and Barb tilted over on a couch, sound asleep.

The man looked down. "I'm sorry to bother you. Paul, the nice young man at the front desk, told me you're a doctor. I'm worried about my wife. She's upstairs in our room, really sick. I was wondering if you could take a look at her."

With trepidation, I followed him upstairs.

Lynn's eyes followed me. She shook her head and said something to Curt.

Before we reached the second floor, Paul followed.

Inside the room, the man's wailing wife rolled on a queen-sized bed. She wailed, and the bedsprings screamed under her weight.

"Blanche. Blanche. Hold still. This nice lady doctor that flew in here on vacation is going to take a look at you."

Blanche stopped rolling and turned to me with a pitiful look, runny mascara, no lipstick, and a butch haircut. Her positive ring sign, with a count of eight rings on her fingers and six piercings in each ear, was complemented with a tattoo on her thigh-sized upper arm. "Up yours."

"What's wrong, Blanche?" I sat down on the bed beside her.

She snarled, "If I knew, I wouldn't be askin' you for help."

Her husband loomed over her. "Enough of that behavior, Blanche. Tell her you're sorry or we are both walking out." He started for the door.

Blanche sat up. "I'm sorry, doctor. I drank a hell of a lot last night. Ate hot salsa and chips, then ended the night with peppermint schnapps to soothe my stomach." She clutched her forehead. "My gut is killing me, and I'm getting a migraine."

We exchanged a few civil questions and answers. After examining her large abdomen and finding a gallbladder scar, I knew it wasn't a gallbladder attack. Based on her history, I suggested her pain could be related to gastritis from too much alcohol and hot salsa. "Blanche, I suggest you sip cold water and chew up a few Rolaids. Then, rest with your head up on three pillows."

"See, Blanche, I told you to try antacids, but no, you had to make me bother the doctor." Her husband pulled a package of Rolaids from the pocket of his baggy Bermuda shorts.

Blanche glared at him and then looked back at me. "We came here on a tour bus. It was a long bumpy ride. I don't think I can stand to get back on that crappy bus this morning. Could we pay you to fly us to Fairbanks?"

The man glared. "Get a grip, Blanche. Don't be such a baby. You're the one who wanted to come here."

I went back downstairs thinking I'd need a cargo plane to carry both of them. The Maule would carry four people, but it is weight limited. The view from the open stairway made the flowered rugs in the lobby look like garden patches, with people taking siestas around the periphery.

The miner hadn't moved, but Color now lay on the couch, curled up by the miner's feet.

Lynn remained at the patient's head, and Curt appeared to be sleeping, his hat over his face.

Ray and Barb had disappeared. The other young miners with Curt sprawled on each end of a long couch, emitting dueling snores.

I sat beside Lynn, waiting in silence and listening to the gurgling sounds from the injured man's throat with no way to clear it. He ground his teeth periodically, making a sickening noise.

Snores of all different rhythms and tunes harmonized around the room. Curt's hat puffed a little with each exhalation.

Finally, in the distance, I heard chopper blades, that wonderful whup-whup-whup.

I poked Lynn's shoulder. "Lynn, do you hear a chopper, or am I hallucinating?"

"I hear it. It must be real if we both hear it."

Paul and I went outside and watched them land in a clearing in front of the hotel, raising a small dust storm in the process. What a wonderful feeling to see the bird settle slowly to the ground. Before the blades stopped, two men in uniform jumped out and turned back toward the door of the aircraft. They pulled out a stretcher with a long board on it and carried it toward the hotel.

"Hi. Fairbanks Rescue Coordination Center said you need a medevac."

I put out my hand in greeting. "Hello, I'm Dr. Kelly McKay. We have a young man with a head injury. Some miners brought him in. Ejected from a single car rollover. One dead at the scene. It happened about midnight. He's been unconscious and decerebrate since he's been here. Quieter the past hour, probably a bad sign. Do you have intubation equipment?"

One of the military men motioned to his partner. "He's got all the drugs and the know-how. Number one flight surgeon at Eielson."

The doctor smiled as they tromped up the steps into the hotel lobby.

The medic started an IV. The doc did a quick survey, palpating everything. Without saying a thing to each other, they went to work, the medic holding the head. The doctor efficiently arranged his intubation tools, pulled out a hand pump suction, and pushed sedating and paralytic drugs IV. The twitching muscles and grinding teeth stopped and the patient's breathing stopped. He was suddenly quiet. His back was no longer arching, his limbs were quiet, and his jaw was slack.

With the military medic holding the head in position, the doctor stretched out on the floor on his belly at the patient's head. He positioned the laryngoscope blade into the patient's mouth and slid the tube in, making it look easy.

I cheered and clapped my hands. "Good job."

He connected oxygen and the resuscitation bag and gave it a few squeezes. The chest wall expanded symmetrically. He listened to the chest and smiled.

The medic assisted in taping the tube securely before placing the patient in a cervical collar. Then we turned and placed him onto the helicopter board and stretcher.

Ray appeared at my side as I was helping.

"Where did you come from? I thought you went to bed."

"Couldn't sleep."

He was a funny man who could rise to an emergency. I thanked him.

Lynn and I watched from the steps as the chopper lifted off from the front of the hotel, sucking up debris and swirling it into the air.

Lynn looked exhausted. "Why don't you just go to bed?"

"I have to sit here and relax. I'll be going to bed soon, after I walk out and tie down the airplane. I was in such a hurry I just left it sitting unsecured. I have to find something to eat, too. Do you want any food?"

She shook her head, "No, I'm not hungry. There isn't any food unless you want to suck on a packet of sugar or have some sweetened coffee."

"That sounds ugly."

". . . and there is no way I'm going to let you go out to the airplane by yourself. Let's scare up a Coke. I'll get us each one."

I agreed.

Lynn returned to the step a few minutes later with two ice-cold Cokes. She sat down beside me.

I told her, "An airplane just landed. I heard him in the pattern when you were inside getting the drinks."

"Enjoy this, Kelly. At two bucks a can, it better be good!"

"Suddenly, I feel exhausted. I can hardly keep my eyes open." I looked back into the lobby through the screen. "There isn't much activity in there. The young miners went back to the mine as soon as Curt saw he wasn't needed. Only Color and George are still here."

I watched a mosquito land on my arm. It tested just where to suck and then filled with red without me even sensing her little needle nose. She flew away, burdened with a heavy red belly.

We walked slowly, silently, down the little road toward the gravel strip. A few bird calls, a periodic irritating mosquito whine, and the crunch of our footsteps broke the silence. About halfway there, Lynn dropped back to pick some flowers. I strolled on.

Sudden crashing, a scream, running footsteps, and a thud.

I spun around in an instant, thinking a moose or some large animal had frightened Lynn.

She lay on the ground not moving. The flowers she had picked were strewn about, and blood was staining her light hair.

A tall man in cutoffs, bare chested with a shaved head, lunged at me. I hit the ground with him on top of me.

I screamed and kicked, trying to get away.

His hand found my mouth and nose. I couldn't breathe. I jerked.

He held me tight.

I was losing consciousness. I could no longer resist. My vision dimmed.

He let go of my mouth and jerked me to my feet by my hair. He drew me closer to him.

I smelled rank breath and body odor. I kicked. My foot struck his crotch.

He screamed and crouched as I backed away out of his reach. "Bitch, you little bitch. After everything I've done for you. You ran away and didn't tell me. I listened to the airplane radio in my room. I heard you tell the controller you were going to Circle. You lied, but I found you anyway."

Keep him talking.

My heart pounded.

The voice, I knew the voice. The voice on the answering machine.

I screamed.

Oh, my God, it was Birdman. I ran.

He caught me, bringing my head under his arm, and dragged me to Lynn. I looked down at her unmoving body.

"I followed you. You stupid bitch. You called the fucking cops on me. I watched you and gave you a little excitement. That streetwalker, beat up and bleeding, made your day at the hospital. I left a couple more for you, but they fought too much. I even signed them, but you didn't catch on. My mark, Birdman wings. But the smart little doctor couldn't figure it out."

He squeezed my head tighter under his arm, making me look down at Lynn.

She's not breathing. He's killed her. I stiffened and stomped on his foot, pulling away.

He tightened his arm around my neck. "I've been following you, keeping track of you. I watched you at the hospital and your apartment. I even left a gift for you there. You didn't say thank you or take me flying. I had to steal a fucking airplane to get here. I can still fly real good."

Birdman grabbed my shoulders.

I kicked and scratched.

"I left other gifts. I thought you'd know it was me. Birdmen like to bring gifts. Birdmen like to fly." He pushed my head down with one hand. "Here is another gift for you. Look at her. Isn't she pretty?" Hyperventilating, he whipped me around to look into his fierce eyes and dragged a small bungie cord out of his dirty shorts. He pushed me to the ground near Lynn and put a foot on my throat. He tried to wrap my hands together. I pushed up on his ankle with both hands, digging my nails into his skin. I twisted and turned. I couldn't breathe. I ripped my nails down his leg.

"Bitch." He stumbled backwards.

I wrenched free and rolled before scrambling to my feet.

He lunged and nearly caught me but landed hard. I didn't look back. I was near the airplane. I ran and ran. I could hear his raspy breathing and swearing.

"Listen to me, you bitch. I thought you were different. I loved you." His voice was too close. I ran faster.

Suddenly he was on me, and I fell, still yards from the plane. He held my long hair again and pulled me up.

His eyes were wild, muscles tense. He pulled me to him and kissed me on the mouth. His khaki shorts bulged in front from his erection. His face and chest had smears of dried blood. He jerked my head down, forcing me to my knees. He exposed himself and pushed my head down, trying to penetrate my mouth.

I smelled rank urine and sweat.

I clenched my teeth.

The penis separated my lips. Gross crystals of urine and rank body fluids entered my mouth.

I gagged. His penis rammed into my mouth.

I crunched down hard.

He jerked my head back and threw me to the ground.

Birdman clutched his genitals. He seethed as I ran. "You're dead, bitch. Just like that friend of yours."

I ran harder, not looking back, and rounded the front of the plane, jumped in, jammed in the key, and hit the starter. I flipped the lock on the passenger door praying the motor would catch on the first try.

The prop didn't catch.

I hit it again.

I looked to see where Birdman was. Close.

The prop sounded like it would catch.

A couple of revolutions.

I gave it more fuel. It coughed, caught, and sounded strong. I jammed in the throttle and careened onto the taxiway just as I heard a crack. The passenger door jerked open.

"Bitch, you fucking bitch. Stop! Get out of the plane!" He hung onto the plane.

I could hardly hear him over the noise of the motor with the door open.

The plane accelerated.

He ran beside the plane, hanging onto the door frame, the strut, being dragged.

I gave it full power and stood on the right rudder peddle. He almost disappeared under the plane as it jerked to the right.

The narrow taxiway forced me to hit the left rudder to bring the plane back.

He gripped the wing strut.

I violently stabbed the left rudder peddle and then the right. Damn, he got a better hold. I dragged him.

I gave it more throttle. The gull-wing door buffeted him as he galloped and dragged with one leg over the landing gear, an arm locked around the bottom of the passenger seat.

Back and forth, back and forth, I rocked the plane, easing off on the throttle to maintain control, and then, just before turning onto the runway, I pushed the throttle in full, accelerating slower than usual.

Faster, faster, come on, faster. Thirty, forty, fifty.

Fly, dammit, fly.

Finally, the tail lifted. Airspeed. Watch the airspeed. Don't crash. Fly the airplane above all else. Listen to Marty's voice. Kelly, fly the airplane.

At sixty-five, I jerked the Maule off the ground, dragging Birdman into the air.

Airborne.

Sixty-five. Climbing. The noise of the engine and the buffeting door was deafening.

Birdman screamed.

The Maule climbed at an awkward angle.

The top of Birdman's shaved head was visible at the seat cushion level. He clung to the seat supports, one leg locked over the wheel strut. The gull-wing door bent in the wind.

I rocked the wings and watched the airspeed indicator.

Marty's voice repeated in my brain, "Remember airspeed control at all times. It's loss of airspeed control that kills people."

Something else was trying to kill me now. His beautiful black curly hair was all gone. His brain function had gone haywire. A serial killer.

Suddenly, Birdman lurched upward and got ahold of the passenger seat.

I struck him with my fist. He groped blindly, trying to get a hold on me. I jerked the plane into a steep bank, throwing the right wing downward, trying to dump him out.

He slipped and nearly disappeared from view.

I remembered the first time I saw him violent in the ER, after he had been so normal at CAP. Vic had warned me, "He's a dangerous man." Vic was right.

Birdman had been killing prey and delivering it to me. He had brought me gifts. He had killed Lynn.

Lynn is dead.

Lynn can't be dead.

Lynn is dead.

I rocked the controls violently and screamed. "You son of a bitch, let go!"

We climbed higher. With him still hanging on, it was very difficult to fly the airplane, to keep it level. At full power, we were only five hundred feet off the ground.

I rocked the plane to the right. Bad mistake. It gave him a better hold. His head came into view again. I saw his hand clutching at the seat bottom.

The sound of the wind was deafening.

I rocked violently to the left, throwing him outward.

He still hung on.

The stall-warning horn blared. I pushed the nose of the plane forward to keep from losing control and stalling.

The airplane shook.

I leveled out the wings and gave it left rudder to counter the weight hanging on the right side and pushed forward to gain speed. The stall warning quit.

Then I climbed to gain more altitude and maneuvering safety, two thousand, three thousand. He still hung on, flying with one leg over the wheel strut and arms clinging to the bottom of the seat.

The wind from the prop and the flying was generating a tremendous force, but Birdman had impressive strength due to his adrenaline surge. Blood vessels bulged on his bloody forehead. I couldn't see his face. I hoped he was tiring. I decided to try another tactic, not giving him time to rest. I rocked the right wing down and then level rather than right wing up, which had almost thrown him into the cockpit the last time.

Down. Level. Down. Level.

I had to be careful. We didn't have a lot of altitude. I still tried to climb, and then I abruptly banked to the left, putting the left wing down sharply. A sixty-degree bank, like in the commercial pilot exam. Hold altitude and hold the steep bank. I looked out the door. Loud wind and motor noise. I pulled back sharply, increasing the g load and making it more difficult for him to hang on.

"Let go, damn you, let go."

Shit, what can I do with this madman killer? I can't shake him off.

I am supposed to save lives, but he'll kill me unless I do something.

I reached into the pocket on the back of the passenger seat. The cold metal of my PPK was there. It was hard to reach, but because I had not put on a seat belt, I was able to stretch my upper body toward it and get a good hold.

I leveled the plane out, and suddenly Birdman was climbing in. His left leg wrapped around the bottom of the seat. His right hand locked on the yoke. He screamed, "Bitch, you bitch, I'll kill you!" He pulled the plane into a near vertical turn to the right. I thought we'd invert.

I hung on and turned back with all my strength. With no seat belt, the force pulled me out of my seat toward the open door. My feet came off the rudder pedals.

Fly the airplane, damn it, Kelly.

Fifty-five, not fifty-six, not fifty-four, fifty-five, damn it, fifty-five.

We were in a spinning dive. I looked at the airspeed.

Near redline. The plane was not designed for this stress.

Any fast moves could rip off a wing.

I pulled myself back down on the seat.

With just one hand, I couldn't resist his pull on the controls. He had us in a death spin.

I emptied all 7 rounds of the PPK into his chest.

The rapid-fire gunshots, muffled by wind and motor, sounded like a pop gun.

His fingers released the yoke.

I dropped the gun in my lap, pulled back power, and flattened the turn.

I pressed on the right rudder to counter the left spin.

His leg caught. He dangled for an instant and then disappeared.

Suddenly, the weight was gone. I had more control of the plane.

Birdman fell.

Birdman flew.

The gull-wing door fluttered and banged.

The world spun slower and slower.

I gently pulled back on the yoke to get out of the deadly turning.

The plane flew easier. The wind noise decreased.

My legs were shaking so much that I took my feet off the rudder pedals and leveled the wings.

The altimeter read 600 feet.

I added power and climbed.

I was finally safe, but my body felt like it was shorting out—exploding.

Gradually, I calmed, and I slowly climbed in a gentle circle

I turned on the GPS to get the coordinates of Birdman's approximate landing site, so I could report it to authorities.

At 5,000 feet, I began calling Fairbanks Radio. At 7,500, they answered.

"Fairbanks Radio, this Maule November Nine One One Delta Romeo. I'm circling over Hot Dam Hot Springs. The hotel radio is still out. They need help right away at the hotel. There has been a murder. Please send help. Send a rescue helicopter. Others may be injured. The killer is dead."

"Yes, ma'am. Troopers and a medical chopper will be dispatched immediately."

I headed back. I spotted Hot Dam and turned toward the runway. The wind noise from the unlatched door was still distracting. I flew a standard pattern.

Marty was in my head. "Set everything up right, every time. Pay attention to the flying,"

I landed, bouncing a couple of times.

It was not my best landing, but I was down. I taxied off the runway and shut down the motor. I sat there shaking and crying.

Ray opened my door.

"It's okay, Kelly. You're going to be all right. You are one helluva pilot."

Barbara was standing a few feet away crying. She grabbed me as soon as I set foot out of the airplane. "We watched you trying to shake that bastard off. He must have been very strong. We thought you were going to crash before he finally let go."

"He wouldn't let go. I shot him."

We walked slowly back toward the hotel, one on each side of me. We walked to the brushy area on the curve where Birdman had jumped Lynn and me. I kneeled beside Lynn's body. A bloody rock lay near her head. Barb said, "Oh, my God, we didn't see her!"

I pressed on Lynn's neck, searching for a carotid pulse. Tears blinded me.

A pulse.

I found a pulse.

I had thought she was dead.

Ray knelt beside me.

"Lynn's alive." I examined her scalp, her neck, and placed my hand on her chest.

Lynn pushed my hand away and kicked one leg,

I positioned her and thrust her jaw forward to open her airway. "Go get some help from the hotel. Some blankets, something stiff to carry her on."

Ray ran toward the hotel.

Barb stayed with me. "After Ray went back to bed, I woke up, and neither one of us could sleep. I wanted to get up and go for a walk. We checked your room and wondered where you were. We were just starting down the road when we heard an airplane engine. It didn't make sense that you'd be flying after such a night. We looked up and saw the airplane barely clear the trees on takeoff, rocking violently, with a guy hanging outside on the passenger door. We broke into a run toward the airstrip."

"Thank you for being here."

"Kelly, you are a damn good pilot. I saw you rock that flying bastard to his death. You're awesome. Remember that."

Lynn moaned. Her eyelids flickered. Some men arrived with the same door the miners had used for the car accident victim.

"What happened?" Lynn looked around, confused.

"Birdman tried to kill us." My voice shook. "Birdman is dead. Now we'll be safe." Ray held me around the shoulders and effused strength into me.

Concerned faces looked down on us.

I stared at them, not really focusing. "A psychotic killer stalked me from Anchorage to Hot Dam. I didn't think anyone except the police knew we were here hiding."

A voice asked, "How did he get here?"

"Stole a Cessna from the Civil Air Patrol in Anchorage where he volunteered. He was a pilot before his psychotic episode a few years ago." Lynn closed her eyes and lay still. Mosquitoes buzzed around us. "I didn't know he was here until he attacked me and my friend Lynn when we were walking out to tie down my airplane. I thought he had killed Lynn."

I rubbed my neck. "He choked me, but I was able to break away and ran to my airplane to get away." I explained the rest. "Thanks for the help. Let's carry Lynn back to the hotel."

Their faces flooded with relief. "How do we get help?"

"After he fell, I contacted Fairbanks by radio. They are sending a trooper and medical helicopter. I wasn't sure if he'd hurt anyone else. I told them one person was dead. I thought he had killed Lynn." I supervised Lynn's move to the door serving as a stretcher and walked with them, holding her head and neck. We placed her on the floor, and I sat beside her, as I had with the man in the vehicular accident.

Barb handed me a cup of strong coffee. She wanted to leave Hot Dam before their scheduled bus trip.

"After we talk to the police and get Lynn en route to the hospital, I'll fly you to Fairbanks, after I take a nap."

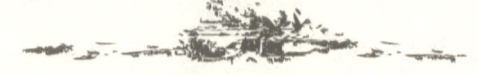

The state trooper arrived by helicopter soon after I had assured myself that Lynn was in good hands with medics from Eielson Air Force Base. The military helicopter provided support to civilians in unusual situations. I guess this situation might be called unusual.

The troopers introduced themselves, but I was so tired and stressed I didn't catch either name. Their interrogation was quick but thorough. I wrote out a report at the breakfast table while fried eggs congealed on my plate. One said, "We got a call from Anchorage reporting the stolen aircraft. I don't think anyone suspected it was someone they knew." He checked my statement. "When I return to Fairbanks, I'll call Detective Moore and tell him what happened up here. I'm really sorry about your friend's injuries. I hope she'll recover."

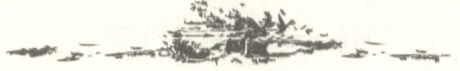

After less than twenty-four hours of friendship with Ray and Barb, I did not want to lose touch with them. I dropped them at the airport in Fairbanks, where we exchanged contact information and promises to meet again someday. I remained at Lynn's bedside in Fairbanks. Her concussion left her with a headache and nausea, but the neurologist released her to me for the flight back to Anchorage.

At Merrill Field, we had no way to get home. I tied down the Maule and called Cornell Ramsey at home. His wife answered. I identified myself and explained the circumstances. "Oh, Kelly, he is so upset. Cornell, Cornell," she called, "It's Dr. McKay. She's back and needs a ride."

He took the phone. "Where are you?"

I told him.

"We're coming to get you. You are coming home with us."

I piled our two small backpacks in front of the plane and sat on them, leaving Lynn sitting in the plane. Cornell got out of his car and held out his hands to help me stand. "Glad you're okay, Kelly. I was so worried." He gave me a long bear-hug. Cornell looked at Lynn. "Let's help her into my car. Does she need to go to the hospital, or can she stay with us?"

"Lynn's stable. She's fine to come with us."

"We found out right after you left that Brett Warren went to drug rehab in Seattle. We didn't know John Reilly might be a killer. We only knew him as a wingnut, never a violent stalker."

Cornell's wife got out of the car. "How are you, Kelly?"

"I'm okay but still in a state of disbelief."

She helped place our packs in the trunk while her husband helped Lynn. "Nice to meet both of you. So sorry this happened."

"Do you want to go pick up some things from your place?"

"I need some clean clothes and a shower."

"Get some clothes for you and Lynn. Shower at our place. I have lasagna in the oven, and Cornell was just mixing a drink."

I adjusted Lynn's seat belt and explained what we were doing. "Sounds good. I just want to sleep. Cornell will keep us safe. We need to be safe. I don't want to die." She closed her eyes.

After dinner, I tucked Lynn in bed. Cornell handed me a Sapphire martini when I came out of the bedroom. I took it in both hands and slurped the icy gin. I cooled my throat, and, sitting in their sunny living room with a view of the Chugach Range, we sipped our drinks. I explained what Birdman had said. The dead girls with bloody carvings on them finally made sense. They were gifts to me from a crazy man, signed with the symbol of a bird's wings.

Chapter 33 Recovery

Lynn's hysterical mother handed the phone to her husband. After I explained the circumstances to the concerned man, he said, "I'll fly in tomorrow to collect Lynn. We'll bring our baby back home." His voice cracked. The line went dead.

I visited Regional ER. It was a teary mess. The staff had recently lost three staff members and nearly lost the two of us. The other physicians begged me to stay, but I wanted to run far away.

"Right now, I need to leave Alaska. I want to return, but I need to put some distance between me and the turmoil."

Vic put his arm around me. I liked his touch and strength. "I wish you wouldn't leave, Kelly. I had some plans for you, some fun. Please come back."

"We may both return, but we need time to recover. I have a friend in Montana who invited us to visit his ranch. I think that will be my first destination. Lynn will be in Boston for a while with her parents."

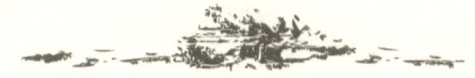

I sold my car, moved out of the apartment, and gave some things to Ed and Lucille and the rest to charity. I put Lynn's clothing and Porsche in storage for her, and then packed what I could carry in the Maule.

It was hard to leave the many close friends I'd developed, but a feeling of doom and the sense of being followed would require time to dissipate.

On my last visit to see Lucille and Ed, I left with a new friend, an eight-week-old blue-eyed sled dog. She curled up on a soft blanket at the bottom of a box strapped in the passenger seat beside me.

On takeoff, her ears perked up, and then she dropped back to sleep for the first leg of her flight to Montana and peace in the Rocky Mountains.

THE END

Questions and Topics for Discussion

1. Did the plot of *Deadly Spin* keep you interested? How did the Alaskan environment contribute to the story?

2. Were the emergency room scenes realistic and understandable? Did they give you a feeling of being there?

3. Two themes in the book are workplace politics (refusing to care for a patient) and unacceptable staff behavior (possible drinking on the job). Would you deal with similar circumstances differently than Kelly did?

4. Have you been confronted with the complexities of unethical and dangerous staff behavior?

5. Did you follow the flying scenes? Were the descriptions clear? Would you like to become a pilot?

6. Did the book end the way you expected?

7. What did you like best about *Deadly Spin*?

8. Are you interested reading the next book, *Deadly Crosswind*, set in Montana?

Afterword

Thank you for reading *DEADLY SPIN*. I hope you enjoyed it. If you did:

- Tell your friends and help others find the book.
- Please write a review at your favorite retail purchase site.
- Like my Facebook page:

  http://www.facebook.com/betty.kuffel

- Visit my website: http://bettykuffel.com

I enjoy discussing my novels with book club readers. If your group is interested in talking with me during your discussion of *DEADLY SPIN*, please contact me at:

MontanaSunriseBooks@gmail.com to schedule a time to Skype.

Betty Kuffel

Acknowledgements

M any thanks to Dennis Foley and friends in Authors of the Flathead who have been instrumental in guiding my writing over years. Special thanks to enduring critique members, Debbie Burke, Deborah Epperson, Marie Martin, Phyllis Quatman, Susan Purvis and Ann Coleman, who remain generous with their time and skills. I also thank my husband Tom for his support and publication formatting, and editor Kathy McKay who provided advice for improving the final product.

About The Author
Betty Kuffel, MD

Dr. Kuffel is a pilot and retired ER physician. The former Alaskan resident lives in Montana. Medical and wilderness experiences, flying, dog sled racing and surviving a plane crash in snowy mountains fuel her writing.

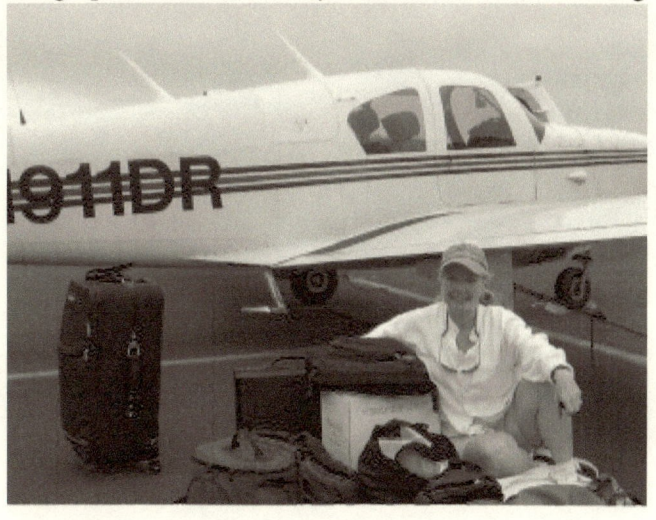